0 POINT WEIGHT LOSS COOKBOOK FOR BEGINNERS

Delicious and Nutritious Dishes to Keep You on Track

Sophia J. Smith

INTRODUCTION

Welcome to the "0 Point Weight Loss Cookbook for Beginners." This book is your guide to enjoying delicious, healthy meals while achieving your weight loss goals effortlessly. The concept of zero-point foods allows you to eat satisfying portions of nutritious foods without the hassle of counting points. Whether you're new to zero-point eating or looking for fresh recipe ideas, this cookbook provides a variety of meals that are easy to prepare and enjoyable to eat.

With a focus on natural, wholesome ingredients, the recipes in this book will help you nourish your body, support your weight loss journey, and develop sustainable, healthy eating habits. From breakfast to dinner, snacks to side dishes, you'll find an array of flavorful options to keep your meals exciting and fulfilling. Let's embark on this journey together and discover how delicious and straightforward healthy eating can be. Enjoy the process, savor the flavors, and celebrate the positive changes in your life.

TABLE OF CONTENTS

Chapter: 1 Breakfast Recipes

1.1 Veggie-Packed Scrambled Eggs

Ingredients

- 4 large eggs
- 1/2 cup diced bell peppers (red, yellow, or green)
- 1/2 cup chopped spinach
- 1/4 cup diced onions
- 1/4 cup diced tomatoes
- 1/4 cup sliced mushrooms
- 1/4 cup low-fat milk (optional for creamier texture)
- Salt and pepper to taste
- 1 tablespoon olive oil or cooking spray

Directions

1. Heat a non-stick skillet over medium heat. Add 1 tablespoon of olive oil or spray with cooking spray.
2. Add 1/4 cup diced onions and 1/2 cup diced bell peppers to the skillet. Sauté for about 3 minutes until they start to soften.
3. Add 1/4 cup sliced mushrooms and cook for another 2 minutes.
4. Stir in 1/4 cup diced tomatoes and 1/2 cup chopped spinach. Cook until the spinach wilts, about 2 minutes.
5. In a bowl, crack 4 large eggs and whisk them together. Add 1/4 cup low-fat milk (optional) for a creamier texture. Season with salt and pepper to taste.
6. Pour the egg mixture over the sautéed vegetables in the skillet.
7. Allow the eggs to set slightly, then gently stir and fold them to combine with the vegetables. Cook until the eggs are fully cooked but still moist, about 3-5 minutes.

8. Transfer the veggie-packed scrambled eggs to a plate and serve hot. Enjoy on their own or with a side of whole-grain toast or avocado slices.

Cooking and Prep Time

Prep Time: 10 minutes

Cook Time: 10 minutes

Total Time: 20 minutes

Serving

Serves 2

Nutrition (per serving)

Calories: 180

Protein: 14g

Carbohydrates: 8g

Dietary Fiber: 2g

Sugars: 4g

Total Fat: 10g

Saturated Fat: 2.5g

Cholesterol: 327mg

Sodium: 180mg

1.2 Berry Smoothie Bowl

Ingredients:

- 1 cup mixed berries (fresh or frozen)
- 1/2 banana, sliced
- 1/2 cup plain Greek yogurt
- 1/4 cup almond milk (or any milk of your choice)
- 1 tablespoon honey (optional, adjust sweetness to taste)
- Toppings (optional): sliced banana, granola, chia seeds, shredded coconut, additional berries

Directions:

1. Blend: Combine mixed berries, sliced banana, Greek yogurt, almond milk, and honey (if using) in a blender.
2. Blend Until Smooth: Blend until smooth and creamy, adjusting the consistency with more almond milk if needed.
3. Serve: Pour the smoothie into a bowl.
4. Add Toppings: Top with sliced banana, granola, chia seeds, shredded coconut, and additional berries as desired.
5. Enjoy: Serve immediately and enjoy your refreshing berry smoothie bowl!

Cooking and Prep Time:

Prep Time: 5 minutes

Cook Time: 0 minutes

Total Time: 5 minutes

Serving:

Serves 1

Nutrition (per serving):

Calories: 300

Protein: 15g

Carbohydrates: 50g

Dietary Fiber: 8g
Sugars: 34g
Total Fat: 5g
Saturated Fat: 1g
Cholesterol: 5mg
Sodium: 100mg

1.3 Greek Yogurt Parfait with Fresh Fruit

Ingredients:

- 1 cup Greek yogurt (plain or flavored)
- 1/2 cup fresh mixed berries (such as strawberries, blueberries, raspberries)
- 1/4 cup granola
- 1 tablespoon honey (optional, for added sweetness)
- Fresh mint leaves (optional, for garnish)

Directions:

1. Layering the Parfait:

- In a serving glass or bowl, start by adding a layer of Greek yogurt.
- Top the yogurt with a layer of fresh mixed berries.
- Sprinkle a layer of granola over the berries.
- Repeat the layers until you reach the top of the glass or bowl, ending with a layer of granola on top.

2. Drizzling with Honey:

- If desired, drizzle honey over the top layer of granola for added sweetness.

3. Garnish (optional):

- Garnish with fresh mint leaves for a pop of color and extra freshness.

4. Serve:

- Serve immediately and enjoy your nutritious and delicious Greek yogurt parfait with fresh fruit!

Cooking and Prep Time:

Prep Time: 5 minutes

Cook Time: 0 minutes

Total Time: 5 minutes

Serving:

Serves 1

Nutrition (per serving):

Calories: 300

Protein: 20g

Carbohydrates: 40g

Dietary Fiber: 5g

Sugars: 20g

Total Fat: 8g

Saturated Fat: 2g

Cholesterol: 10mg

Sodium: 100mg

1.4 Oatmeal with Apple and Cinnamon

Ingredients:

Oatmeal:

- 1/2 cup old fashioned rolled oats
- 1 cup water or milk
- 1/2 Tablespoon maple syrup, brown sugar or coconut sugar (optional)
- 1/4-1/2 teaspoon ground cinnamon
- 1/2 teaspoon vanilla extract
- Pinch of sea salt
- 2 Tablespoons chopped pecans, for topping

Cinnamon Apples:

- 1/2 cup diced apples
- 2 teaspoons maple syrup
- 1/4 teaspoon cinnamon

Instructions:

1. In a small saucepan, sauté the diced apples, maple syrup and cinnamon for a few minutes until the apples are soft and caramelized. Set aside.
2. Add the oats, water, maple syrup, cinnamon, vanilla and salt to a saucepan over medium-high heat. Bring the mixture to a low boil, then reduce heat to a low simmer and cook for 5-7 minutes, stirring occasionally, until the oats have soaked up most of the liquid and are creamy.
3. Transfer the oatmeal to a bowl and top with the cinnamon apples, pecans, a sprinkle of cinnamon and additional sweetener if desired.

Prep Time: 3 minutes

Cook Time: 7 minutes

Total Time: 10 minutes

Servings: 1

Nutrition (per serving):

Calories: 361

Carbohydrates: 50g

Protein: 9g

Fat: 13g

Saturated Fat: 1g

Sodium: 472mg

Potassium: 418mg

Fiber: 9g

Sugar: 14g

1.5 Spinach and Mushroom Breakfast Wrap

Ingredients:

- 4 large eggs
- 1 tablespoon olive oil
- 1/4 cup diced onion
- 1 cup sliced mushrooms
- 1 1/2 cups fresh baby spinach
- 1/4 teaspoon salt
- 1/8 teaspoon black pepper
- 4 whole wheat tortilla wraps

Instructions:

1. In a medium skillet, heat the olive oil over medium heat. Add the diced onion and sauté for 2-3 minutes until translucent.
2. Add the sliced mushrooms to the skillet and continue cooking for 3-4 minutes, until the mushrooms are softened.
3. In a small bowl, beat the eggs with the salt and pepper.
4. Push the onions and mushrooms to the side of the skillet, then pour the beaten eggs into the empty side. Let the eggs cook for 30 seconds to 1 minute, then gently stir to scramble them.
5. Once the eggs are cooked through, stir in the fresh spinach and continue cooking for 1-2 minutes until the spinach is wilted.
6. Divide the egg, spinach, and mushroom mixture evenly among the 4 tortilla wraps. Fold the wraps and enjoy!

Prep and Cook Time:

- Prep Time: 10 minutes
- Cook Time: 15 minutes
- Total Time: 25 minutes

Serving and Nutrition:

This recipe makes 4 breakfast wraps. Each wrap contains:

- Calories: 246
- Total Fat: 11g
- Saturated Fat: 3g
- Cholesterol: 226mg
- Sodium: 658mg
- Total Carbohydrates: 25g
- Fiber: 1g
- Sugar: 1g
- Protein: 13g

1.6 Egg White and Veggie Frittata

Ingredients:

- 1 tablespoon olive oil
- 1 red bell pepper, diced
- 1 cup cherry tomatoes, halved
- 2 cloves garlic, minced
- 2 cups baby spinach, chopped
- 1 1/2 cups egg whites (about 6 large eggs' worth)
- 1/4 teaspoon salt
- 1/8 teaspoon black pepper
- 1/2 cup crumbled feta cheese (optional)

Instructions:

1. Preheat oven to 400°F. Grease a 9-inch pie dish or oven-safe skillet with olive oil.
2. In a skillet over medium heat, heat the olive oil. Add the diced bell pepper and sauté for 3-4 minutes until starting to soften.
3. Add the cherry tomatoes and garlic to the skillet. Cook for 2 more minutes until tomatoes are slightly blistered.
4. Add the chopped spinach to the skillet and cook for 1 minute until wilted. Remove from heat.
5. In a medium bowl, whisk together the egg whites, salt and pepper.
6. Spread the vegetable mixture evenly in the prepared pie dish or skillet. Pour the egg white mixture over top.
7. Bake for 25-30 minutes, until the egg whites are set.
8. Remove from oven and let cool for 5 minutes. Slice and serve warm, optionally topped with crumbled feta cheese.

Cooking Time:

- Prep Time: 10 minutes

- Cook Time: 30 minutes
- Total Time: 40 minutes

Serving and Nutrition:

This recipe makes 4-6 servings, depending on how you slice it. Each serving contains:

- Calories: 100
- Total Fat: 3g
- Saturated Fat: 1g
- Cholesterol: 0mg
- Sodium: 400mg
- Total Carbohydrates: 7g
- Fiber: 2g
- Sugar: 4g
- Protein: 13g

1.7 Avocado and Tomato Toast

Ingredients:

- 2 slices bread
- 1 ripe avocado
- 6 cherry tomatoes, halved
- 1 teaspoon balsamic vinegar
- Salt and pepper, to taste
- Extra virgin olive oil (optional)

Instructions:

1. **Toast the Bread**: Toast the bread slices in a toaster until golden brown.
2. **Prepare the Avocado**: Halve and pit the avocado. Scoop the flesh into a bowl and mash. Mix in a squeeze of lemon juice and season with salt and pepper to taste.
3. **Assemble the Toast**:
   - Spread the avocado mixture evenly onto the toasted bread.
   - Arrange the halved cherry tomatoes on top of the avocado.
   - Drizzle with balsamic vinegar and a light sprinkle of salt and pepper.
   - Optionally, add a drizzle of extra virgin olive oil for extra flavor.
4.

Cooking Time:

- **Prep Time**: 5 minutes
- **Cook Time**: 5 minutes
- **Total Time**: 10 minutes

Serving and Nutrition:

This recipe makes 2 servings. Each serving contains:

- **Calories**: 267
- **Total Fat**: 22g

- **Saturated Fat**: 3g
- **Cholesterol**: 0mg
- **Sodium**: 150mg
- **Total Carbohydrates**: 24g
- **Fiber**: 6g
- **Sugar**: 2g
- **Protein**: 3g

1.8 Cottage Cheese with Pineapple

Ingredients:

- 16 oz cottage cheese, low-fat or non-fat
- 10 oz canned pineapple chunks, drained
- 1 tsp chia seeds (optional)
- Mint leaves for garnish (optional)
- Maple syrup (optional)

Instructions:

1. In a medium bowl or individual serving containers, layer the cottage cheese and pineapple chunks.
2. Top with chia seeds, if using, and a few mint leaves for garnish.
3. Drizzle with a small amount of maple syrup, if desired.
4. Serve immediately or refrigerate until ready to enjoy.

Cooking Time:

- Prep Time: 5 minutes
- Total Time: 5 minutes

Serving and Nutrition:

This recipe makes 2-3 servings, depending on portion size.

Nutrition per serving (based on 3 servings):

- Calories: 167
- Total Fat: 3g
- Saturated Fat: 2g
- Cholesterol: 12mg
- Sodium: 338mg
- Total Carbohydrates: 19g
- Fiber: 2g
- Sugars: 15g

1.9 Green Protein Smoothie

Ingredients:

- 1 frozen banana
- 1 scoop vanilla protein powder
- 1 cup unsweetened almond milk (or milk of choice)
- 2 cups baby spinach, loosely packed
- 1 tablespoon chia seeds

Instructions:

1. Place all ingredients into a high-powered blender.
2. Blend on high until smooth and creamy.

Cooking Time:

- Prep Time: 5 minutes
- Total Time: 5 minutes

Serving and Nutrition:

This recipe makes 1 serving. The nutrition information is as follows:

- Calories: 268
- Total Carbohydrates: 38g
- Protein: 17g
- Fat: 8g
- Fiber: 11g
- Sugar: 15g

1.10 Banana Oat Pancakes

Ingredients:

- 2 medium ripe bananas
- 2 eggs
- 1/2 cup unsweetened almond milk (or milk of choice)
- 1 teaspoon vanilla extract
- 1 1/2 cups old-fashioned rolled oats
- 2 teaspoons baking powder
- 1/4 teaspoon salt
- Butter or oil for cooking

Instructions:

1. Add the bananas, eggs, almond milk, and vanilla to a blender. Blend on high until smooth.
2. Add the rolled oats, baking powder, and salt to the blender. Blend again until the batter is well combined and the oats are finely ground.
3. Heat a large non-stick skillet or griddle over medium heat. Grease with a small amount of butter or oil.
4. Scoop the batter onto the hot surface, using about 1/4 cup for each pancake. Cook for 2-3 minutes per side, until golden brown.
5. Serve the banana oat pancakes warm, with desired toppings such as fresh fruit, maple syrup, nut butter, or yogurt.

Cooking Time:

- Prep Time: 5 minutes
- Cook Time: 10-15 minutes
- Total Time: 15-20 minute

Serving and Nutrition:

This recipe makes approximately 8-10 pancakes, depending on size. Each serving (2-3 pancakes) contains:

- Calories: 250
- Total Fat: 7g
- Saturated Fat: 2g
- Cholesterol: 95mg
- Sodium: 380mg
- Total Carbohydrates: 38g
- Fiber: 5g
- Sugars: 12g
- Protein: 9g

1.11 Baked Tomato and Basil Eggs

Ingredients:

- 4 medium tomatoes, halved
- 4-5 fresh basil leaves, chopped
- 4 large eggs
- 1/2 teaspoon salt
- 1/2 teaspoon black pepper
- 2 tablespoons olive oil
- 2 cloves garlic, sliced
- 1/4 cup grated Parmesan cheese
- 2 tablespoons heavy cream or milk

Instructions:

1. Preheat the oven to 400°F (200°C).
2. Arrange the tomato halves in a shallow baking dish. Sprinkle the chopped basil over the tomatoes.
3. Crack the eggs into the spaces between the tomato halves. Season with salt and pepper.
4. In a small bowl, mix together the olive oil, sliced garlic, Parmesan cheese, and heavy cream or milk. Pour this mixture over the eggs and tomatoes.
5. Bake for 20-25 minutes, or until the eggs are set and the tomatoes are softened.
6. Serve the baked tomato and basil eggs warm, garnished with additional fresh basil if desired.

Cooking Time:

- Prep Time: 10 minutes
- Cook Time: 20-25 minutes
- Total Time: 30-35 minutes

Serving and Nutrition:

This recipe makes 4 servings. Each serving contains:

- Calories: 180
- Total Fat: 13g
- Saturated Fat: 4g
- Cholesterol: 215mg
- Sodium: 480mg
- Total Carbohydrates: 7g
- Fiber: 2g
- Sugars: 5g
- Protein: 11g

1.12 Apple Cinnamon Yogurt Bowl

Ingredients:

- 1 apple, peeled, cored and diced
- 1 tablespoon maple syrup
- 1/2 teaspoon ground cinnamon
- 1/4 teaspoon ground nutmeg
- 1 cup plain Greek yogurt
- 1/4 cup granola

Instructions:

1. In a small saucepan, combine the diced apple, maple syrup, cinnamon and nutmeg. Cook over medium heat for 4-5 minutes, stirring occasionally, until the apples are softened.
2. Remove the apple mixture from heat and let cool slightly.
3. In a bowl, layer the yogurt and apple mixture. Top with granola.
4. Serve immediately.

Cooking Time:

- Prep Time: 5 minutes
- Cook Time: 5 minutes
- Total Time: 10 minutes

Serving and Nutrition:

This recipe makes 1 serving. The nutrition information is as follows:

- Calories: 350
- Total Fat: 5g
- Saturated Fat: 1g
- Cholesterol: 15mg
- Sodium: 100mg
- Total Carbohydrates: 60g

- Fiber: 5g
- Sugars: 40g
- Protein: 20g

1.13 Veggie Breakfast Tacos

Ingredients:

- 2 teaspoons olive oil
- 1 small white or yellow onion, diced
- 3 garlic cloves, minced
- 1 small zucchini, sliced into thin strips
- 1 small yellow squash, sliced into thin strips
- 1 red bell pepper, seeded and chopped
- 1/2 lime, juiced
- Salt and red pepper flakes to taste
- 6 large eggs, scrambled
- Hot sauce (optional)
- 6 small corn or flour tortillas
- 1 jalapeño, seeded and minced (optional)
- 1/4 cup crumbled feta cheese
- Chopped fresh cilantro

Instructions:

1. In a large skillet, heat the olive oil over medium heat. Add the onion and a pinch of salt. Cook for 5 minutes until softened.
2. Add the garlic and a pinch of red pepper flakes. Cook for 30 seconds until fragrant.
3. Add the zucchini, yellow squash, and bell pepper. Cook for 7-8 minutes, stirring occasionally, until the vegetables are tender but still have some bite.
4. Remove the pan from heat and squeeze the lime juice over the vegetable mixture. Season with salt to taste.
5. In a separate skillet, scramble the eggs over medium-low heat until lightly set. Season with salt and pepper.
6. Warm the tortillas according to package instructions.

7. To assemble the tacos, divide the vegetable mixture and scrambled eggs evenly among the tortillas. Top with jalapeño, feta cheese, and chopped cilantro.

8. Serve immediately, with hot sauce on the side if desired.

Cooking Time:

- Prep Time: 15 minutes
- Cook Time: 20 minutes
- Total Time: 35 minutes

Serving and Nutrition:

This recipe makes 6 tacos, with 1 taco per serving. Each serving contains:

- Calories: 280
- Total Fat: 14g
- Saturated Fat: 4g
- Cholesterol: 215mg
- Sodium: 420mg
- Total Carbohydrates: 27g
- Fiber: 5g
- Sugars: 5g
- Protein: 14g

1.14 Chia Seed Breakfast Pudding

Ingredients:

- 3 tablespoons chia seeds
- 1 cup milk (dairy, almond, oat, etc.)
- 1 tablespoon maple syrup (or honey)
- 1/4 teaspoon vanilla extract (optional)
- Toppings of your choice (berries, granola, nuts, etc.)

Instructions:

1. In a medium bowl or mason jar, combine the chia seeds, milk, maple syrup, and vanilla (if using). Stir well to combine.
2. Cover and refrigerate for at least 4 hours, or overnight. Stir the mixture occasionally to prevent clumping.
3. Once the pudding has thickened to your desired consistency, transfer it to serving bowls or jars.
4. Top with your favorite toppings, such as fresh berries, chopped nuts, granola, or a drizzle of nut butter.

Cooking Time:

- Prep Time: 5 minutes
- Chilling Time: 4 hours to overnight
- Total Time: 4 hours 5 minutes to overnight

Serving and Nutrition:

This recipe makes 2 servings. Each serving contains:

- Calories: 170
- Total Fat: 9g
- Saturated Fat: 1g
- Cholesterol: 0mg
- Sodium: 91mg

- Total Carbohydrates: 16g
- Fiber: 13g
- Sugars: 3g
- Protein: 7g

1.15 Fresh Fruit Salad with Mint

Ingredients:

- 1 cup diced pineapple
- 1 cup diced mango
- 1 cup halved strawberries
- 1 cup blueberries
- 1 cup diced kiwi
- 2 tablespoons fresh lime juice
- 1 tablespoon honey
- 1/4 cup chopped fresh mint leaves

Instructions:

1. In a large bowl, combine the diced pineapple, mango, strawberries, blueberries, and kiwi.
2. In a small bowl, whisk together the lime juice and honey to make the dressing.
3. Pour the dressing over the fruit and gently toss to coat evenly.
4. Sprinkle the chopped fresh mint leaves over the top of the fruit salad.
5. Serve immediately or refrigerate until ready to serve.

Cooking Time:

- Prep Time: 15 minutes
- Total Time: 15 minutes

Serving and Nutrition:

This recipe makes 4 servings. Each serving contains:

- Calories: 135
- Total Fat: 1g
- Saturated Fat: 0g
- Cholesterol: 0mg
- Sodium: 2mg

- Total Carbohydrates: 34g
- Fiber: 5g
- Sugars: 27g
- Protein: 2g

Chapter:2 Lunch Recipes

2.1 Grilled Chicken Salad with Lemon Vinaigrette

Ingredients:

For the Lemon Vinaigrette/Marinade:

- 1/3 cup extra virgin olive oil
- 2 tablespoons champagne vinegar or white wine vinegar
- 2 tablespoons fresh lemon juice
- 2 tablespoons honey
- 1 shallot, minced

For the Salad:

- 6 cups mixed salad greens
- 1 pound boneless, skinless chicken breasts
- 1 cup fresh blueberries
- 1/2 cup crumbled feta cheese

Instructions:

1. **Make the Vinaigrette/Marinade:** In a small bowl, whisk together the olive oil, vinegar, lemon juice, honey, and minced shallot until emulsified.
2. **Marinate the Chicken:** Place the chicken breasts in a shallow dish and pour 1/4 cup of the vinaigrette over them, turning to coat both sides. Cover and refrigerate for 30 minutes to 1 hour.
3. **Grill the Chicken:** Preheat a grill or grill pan to medium-high heat. Grill the chicken for 5-7 minutes per side, until cooked through. Allow to rest for 5 minutes, then slice or chop the chicken.

4. **Assemble the Salad:** In a large bowl, toss the mixed greens with 1/4 cup of the remaining vinaigrette. Transfer the dressed greens to a serving platter or individual plates.

5. **Top the Salad:** Arrange the grilled chicken slices, fresh blueberries, and crumbled feta cheese over the greens.

6. **Serve:** Drizzle the remaining vinaigrette over the top of the salad, if desired. Serve immediately.

Cooking Time:

- Prep Time: 15 minutes
- Marinating Time: 30 minutes to 1 hour
- Cook Time: 10-14 minutes
- Total Time: 55 minutes to 1 hour 25 minutes

Serving and Nutrition:

This recipe makes 4 servings. Each serving contains:

- Calories: 390
- Total Fat: 22g
- Saturated Fat: 5g
- Cholesterol: 95mg
- Sodium: 430mg
- Total Carbohydrates: 18g
- Fiber: 3g
- Sugars: 13g
- Protein: 35g

2.2 Veggie Stir-Fry with Tofu

Ingredients:

- 1 block (14 oz) extra-firm tofu, pressed and cubed
- 2 tablespoons cornstarch
- 2 tablespoons sesame oil, divided
- 1 red bell pepper, sliced
- 1 cup broccoli florets
- 1 cup sliced mushrooms
- 3 cloves garlic, minced
- 1 tablespoon grated ginger
- 2 tablespoons soy sauce
- 1 tablespoon rice vinegar
- 1 teaspoon honey
- 1/4 teaspoon red pepper flakes (optional)
- 2 green onions, sliced
- Sesame seeds for garnish

Instructions:

1. **Press the tofu**: Wrap the tofu block in paper towels or a clean kitchen towel. Place a heavy object, like a cast iron skillet, on top and let sit for 15-30 minutes to remove excess moisture.
2. **Prepare the tofu**: Cut the pressed tofu into 1-inch cubes. Place the tofu cubes in a bowl and toss with cornstarch until evenly coated.
3. **Cook the tofu**: Heat 1 tablespoon of sesame oil in a large skillet or wok over medium-high heat. Add the tofu cubes in a single layer and cook for 2-3 minutes per side until crispy and golden brown. Transfer the crispy tofu to a plate and set aside.

4. **Stir-fry the veggies**: In the same skillet, heat the remaining 1 tablespoon of sesame oil over medium-high heat. Add the bell pepper, broccoli, and mushrooms. Stir-fry for 3-4 minutes until the vegetables are tender-crisp.

5. **Add the sauce**: Push the vegetables to the sides of the skillet. Add the garlic and ginger to the center and cook for 30 seconds until fragrant. Whisk together the soy sauce, rice vinegar, honey, and red pepper flakes (if using). Pour the sauce into the skillet and let it simmer for 1-2 minutes.

6. **Finish the dish**: Add the crispy tofu back to the skillet and toss everything together until well combined and heated through. Remove from heat and stir in the sliced green onions.

7. **Serve**: Transfer the veggie stir-fry to a serving bowl or plate. Garnish with sesame seeds. Serve immediately over rice or noodles.

Cooking Time:

- Prep Time: 15 minutes
- Cook Time: 15 minutes
- Total Time: 30 minutes

Serving and Nutrition:

This recipe makes 4 servings. Each serving contains approximately:

- Calories: 250
- Total Fat: 14g
- Saturated Fat: 2g
- Cholesterol: 0mg
- Sodium: 590mg
- Total Carbohydrates: 20g
- Fiber: 5g
- Sugars: 5g
- Protein: 16g

2.3 Tomato Basil Soup

Ingredients:

- 2½ pounds roma tomatoes, halved
- ¼ cup extra-virgin olive oil
- Sea salt and freshly ground black pepper
- 1 medium yellow onion, chopped
- ⅓ cup chopped carrots
- 4 garlic cloves, chopped
- 3 cups vegetable broth
- 1 tablespoon balsamic vinegar
- 1 teaspoon fresh thyme leaves
- 1 loosely packed cup fresh basil leaves, plus more for garnish

Instructions:

1. **Preheat the Oven**: Preheat the oven to 350°F (180°C). Line a baking sheet with parchment paper.
2. **Roast the Tomatoes**: Arrange the halved tomatoes, cut-side up, on the prepared baking sheet. Drizzle with olive oil and season with salt and pepper. Roast for 1 hour, or until the tomatoes are still juicy but starting to shrivel.
3. **Sauté the Aromatics**: In a large pot, heat 1 tablespoon of olive oil over medium heat. Add the chopped onion and cook for 5 minutes until translucent. Add the chopped carrots and cook for another 5 minutes until they start to soften.
4. **Add the Garlic**: Add the chopped garlic and cook for 30 seconds until fragrant.
5. **Simmer the Soup**: Add the roasted tomatoes, vegetable broth, balsamic vinegar, and thyme leaves to the pot. Bring to a boil, then reduce the heat to a simmer. Cook for 20 minutes, or until the flavors have melded together.
6. **Blend the Soup**: Allow the soup to cool slightly. Transfer it to a blender and puree until smooth. Alternatively, use an immersion blender to puree the soup directly in the pot.

7. **Add the Basil**: Add the fresh basil leaves to the blended soup and pulse until just combined.

8. **Season and Serve**: Season the soup with salt and pepper to taste. Serve immediately, garnished with fresh basil leaves and a drizzle of olive oil if desired.

Cooking Time:

- **Prep Time**: 15 minutes
- **Roasting Time**: 1 hour
- **Cooking Time**: 30 minutes
- **Total Time**: 1 hour 45 minutes

Serving and Nutrition:

This recipe makes 4 servings. Each serving contains approximately:

- **Calories**: 250
- **Total Fat**: 14g
- **Saturated Fat**: 2g
- **Cholesterol**: 0mg
- **Sodium**: 590mg
- **Total Carbohydrates**: 20g
- **Fiber**: 5g
- **Sugars**: 5g
- **Protein**: 16g

2.4 Zucchini Noodles with Pesto

Ingredients:

- 3 medium zucchini, spiralized or julienned into noodles
- 1/2 cup basil pesto (homemade or store-bought)
- 2 tablespoons toasted pine nuts or walnuts
- 1/4 cup grated Parmesan cheese (optional)
- Salt and pepper to taste

Instructions:

1. **Prepare the Zucchini Noodles**: Use a spiralizer, julienne peeler, or sharp knife to cut the zucchini into long, thin noodle-like strips.
2. **Cook the Zucchini Noodles**: In a large skillet or wok, heat the zucchini noodles over medium heat for 2-3 minutes, just until they start to soften slightly. Be careful not to overcook them, as you want them to retain some crunch.
3. **Toss with Pesto**: Remove the zucchini noodles from heat and toss them with the basil pesto until evenly coated.
4. **Add Toppings**: Top the pesto zucchini noodles with the toasted pine nuts or walnuts and grated Parmesan cheese (if using).
5. **Season and Serve**: Season with salt and pepper to taste. Serve immediately while the noodles are still warm.

Cooking Time:

- Prep Time: 10 minutes
- Cook Time: 3-5 minutes
- Total Time: 13-15 minutes

Serving and Nutrition:

This recipe makes 2-3 servings, depending on portion size.

Nutrition per serving (based on 3 servings):

- Calories: 170
- Total Fat: 14g
- Saturated Fat: 3g
- Cholesterol: 5mg
- Sodium: 290mg
- Total Carbohydrates: 8g
- Fiber: 2g
- Sugars: 4g
- Protein: 6g

2.5 Chickpea and Avocado Salad

Ingredients:

- 1 (15 oz) can chickpeas, drained and rinsed
- 1 ripe avocado, diced
- 1/2 cup chopped fresh basil
- 1/4 cup chopped red onion
- 1 tablespoon fresh lemon juice
- 1 tablespoon extra-virgin olive oil
- 1/4 teaspoon salt
- 1/8 teaspoon black pepper

Instructions:

1. In a medium bowl, gently mash the chickpeas with a fork or potato masher, leaving some whole chickpeas.
2. Add the diced avocado, chopped basil, red onion, lemon juice, olive oil, salt, and pepper. Stir to combine.
3. Taste and adjust seasoning as needed. Serve immediately or refrigerate until ready to serve.

Cooking Time:

- Prep Time: 10 minutes
- Total Time: 10 minutes

Serving and Nutrition:

This recipe makes 2-3 servings, depending on portion size.

Nutrition per serving (based on 3 servings):

- Calories: 220
- Total Fat: 14g
- Saturated Fat: 2g

- Cholesterol: 0mg
- Sodium: 320mg
- Total Carbohydrates: 20g
- Fiber: 7g
- Sugars: 2g
- Protein: 6g

2.6 Mediterranean Quinoa Salad

Ingredients:

- 1 cup uncooked quinoa, rinsed
- 1 1/2 cups vegetable or chicken broth
- 1 cup cherry tomatoes, halved
- 1 cucumber, diced
- 1/2 cup kalamata olives, halved
- 1/2 cup crumbled feta cheese
- 1/4 cup chopped fresh parsley
- 2 tablespoons chopped fresh basil
- 2 tablespoons olive oil
- 2 tablespoons lemon juice
- 1 garlic clove, minced
- 1/4 teaspoon salt
- 1/4 teaspoon black pepper

Instructions:

1. In a medium saucepan, combine the quinoa and broth. Bring to a boil, then reduce heat to low, cover and simmer for 15-20 minutes, until quinoa is tender and liquid is absorbed. Fluff with a fork and let cool.
2. In a large bowl, combine the cooked quinoa, cherry tomatoes, cucumber, olives, feta, parsley, and basil.
3. In a small bowl, whisk together the olive oil, lemon juice, garlic, salt, and pepper.
4. Pour the dressing over the quinoa salad and toss gently to coat.
5. Serve immediately or refrigerate until ready to serve. The salad can be made up to 3 days in advance.

Cooking Time:

- Prep Time: 15 minutes

- Cook Time: 20 minutes
- Total Time: 35 minutes

Serving and Nutrition:

This recipe makes 4-6 servings, depending on portion size.

Nutrition per serving (based on 4 servings):

- Calories: 280
- Total Fat: 15g
- Saturated Fat: 4g
- Cholesterol: 15mg
- Sodium: 520mg
- Total Carbohydrates: 28g
- Fiber: 4g
- Sugars: 3g
- Protein: 9g

2.7 Black Bean and Corn Salad

Ingredients:

- 1 (15 oz) can black beans, drained and rinsed
- 1 (15 oz) can corn kernels, drained
- 1 red bell pepper, diced
- 1 cup cherry tomatoes, halved
- 1/2 red onion, diced
- 1/4 cup chopped fresh cilantro
- 2 tablespoons lime juice
- 1 tablespoon olive oil
- 1 teaspoon ground cumin
- 1/4 teaspoon chili powder
- Salt and black pepper to taste

Instructions:

1. In a large bowl, combine the drained and rinsed black beans, drained corn kernels, diced red bell pepper, halved cherry tomatoes, and diced red onion.
2. In a small bowl, whisk together the lime juice, olive oil, cumin, chili powder, and a pinch of salt and pepper.
3. Pour the dressing over the bean and vegetable mixture and toss gently to coat everything evenly.
4. Stir in the chopped fresh cilantro.
5. Taste and adjust seasoning as needed, adding more salt, pepper, lime juice, or spices to your preference.
6. Serve immediately or refrigerate until ready to serve. The salad can be made up to 3 days in advance.

Cooking Time:

- Prep Time: 15 minutes

- Total Time: 15 minutes

Serving and Nutrition:

This recipe makes 4-6 servings, depending on portion size.

Nutrition per serving (based on 4 servings):

- Calories: 200
- Total Fat: 6g
- Saturated Fat: 1g
- Cholesterol: 0mg
- Sodium: 320mg
- Total Carbohydrates: 30g
- Fiber: 8g
- Sugars: 5g
- Protein: 8g

2.8 Lettuce Wrap Tacos

Ingredients:

For the Tacos:

- 1 head of romaine lettuce, leaves separated
- 1 pound ground turkey or chicken breast
- 1 medium onion, diced
- 2 cloves garlic, minced
- 1 can (15 oz) black beans, drained and rinsed
- 1 cup cherry tomatoes, halved
- 1 cup shredded cheddar cheese
- 1 cup crumbled feta cheese
- 1/4 cup chopped fresh cilantro
- 1/4 cup chopped fresh parsley
- 1/4 cup chopped fresh dill
- 2 tablespoons olive oil
- 2 tablespoons lime juice
- 1 teaspoon ground cumin
- 1/2 teaspoon chili powder
- Salt and black pepper to taste

For the Toppings:

- Sliced avocado
- Sliced red onion
- Shredded lettuce
- Sliced jalapeño (optional)
- Sliced lime (optional)

Instructions:

1. **Cook the Ground Meat:** In a large skillet, cook the ground turkey or chicken breast over medium-high heat until browned. Break it up into small pieces as it cooks.
2. **Add the Onions and Garlic:** Add the diced onion and minced garlic to the skillet. Cook until the onion is translucent.
3. **Add the Black Beans:** Add the drained and rinsed black beans to the skillet. Cook for 2-3 minutes until they are heated through.
4. **Add the Tomatoes and Cheese:** Add the halved cherry tomatoes and shredded cheddar cheese to the skillet. Cook for 1-2 minutes until the cheese is melted.
5. **Season and Mix:** Add the cumin, chili powder, salt, and black pepper to the skillet. Stir to combine. Remove from heat.
6. **Assemble the Tacos:** Place a lettuce leaf on a plate. Spoon a portion of the ground meat mixture onto the lettuce leaf. Top with sliced avocado, sliced red onion, shredded lettuce, sliced jalapeño (if using), and sliced lime (if using).
7. **Serve:** Repeat with the remaining ingredients to make additional tacos. Serve immediately.

Cooking Time:

- **Prep Time:** 15 minutes
- **Cook Time:** 15 minutes
- **Total Time:** 30 minutes

Serving and Nutrition:

This recipe makes 4-6 servings, depending on portion size.

Nutrition per serving (based on 6 servings):

- **Calories:** 250
- **Total Fat:** 14g
- **Saturated Fat:** 4g
- **Cholesterol:** 30mg
- **Sodium:** 320mg

- **Total Carbohydrates:** 20g
- **Fiber:** 5g
- **Sugars:** 5g
- **Protein:** 20g

2.9 Cucumber and Tomato Gazpacho

Ingredients:

- 2 large cucumbers, peeled, seeded and diced
- 3 large tomatoes, diced
- 1 red onion, diced
- 2 cloves garlic, minced
- 1/4 cup olive oil
- 2 tablespoons red wine vinegar
- 1 tablespoon fresh lime juice
- 1 teaspoon salt
- 1/2 teaspoon black pepper
- 1/4 cup chopped fresh basil
- 1/4 cup chopped fresh parsley

Instructions:

1. In a large bowl, combine the diced cucumbers, tomatoes, red onion, and garlic.
2. In a small bowl, whisk together the olive oil, red wine vinegar, lime juice, salt, and black pepper.
3. Pour the dressing over the vegetable mixture and stir gently to combine.
4. Stir in the chopped basil and parsley.
5. Cover and refrigerate for at least 2 hours, or up to 24 hours, to allow the flavors to meld.
6. Ladle the gazpacho into bowls and serve chilled.

Cooking Time:

- Prep Time: 20 minutes
- Chilling Time: 2-24 hours
- Total Time: 2-24 hours 20 minutes

Serving and Nutrition:

This recipe makes 4-6 servings, depending on portion size.

Nutrition per serving (based on 6 servings):

- Calories: 140
- Total Fat: 10g
- Saturated Fat: 1.5g
- Cholesterol: 0mg
- Sodium: 450mg
- Total Carbohydrates: 12g
- Fiber: 3g
- Sugars: 6g
- Protein: 2g

2.10 Spicy Cauliflower Tacos

Ingredients:

- 1 head of cauliflower, cut into bite-sized florets
- 2 tablespoons olive oil
- 1 teaspoon chili powder
- 1 teaspoon cumin
- 1/2 teaspoon garlic powder
- 1/4 teaspoon cayenne pepper (or more to taste)
- Salt and pepper to taste
- 8-10 small corn or flour tortillas, warmed

Toppings:

- Shredded cabbage or lettuce
- Diced avocado
- Chopped cilantro
- Crumbled queso fresco or feta cheese
- Lime wedges

Instructions:

1. Preheat the oven to 400°F (200°C).
2. In a large bowl, toss the cauliflower florets with the olive oil, chili powder, cumin, garlic powder, cayenne, salt, and pepper until evenly coated.
3. Spread the seasoned cauliflower in a single layer on a baking sheet. Roast for 20-25 minutes, flipping halfway, until the cauliflower is tender and lightly browned.
4. Remove the roasted cauliflower from the oven and let it cool slightly.
5. To assemble the tacos, place a spoonful of the spicy roasted cauliflower in the center of a warm tortilla. Top with shredded cabbage or lettuce, diced avocado, chopped cilantro, and crumbled queso fresco or feta cheese.

6. Serve the tacos immediately, with lime wedges on the side for squeezing over the top.

Cooking Time:

- Prep Time: 10 minutes
- Cook Time: 20-25 minutes
- Total Time: 30-35 minutes

Serving and Nutrition:

This recipe makes 8-10 tacos, depending on the size of the tortillas and how much filling is used per taco.

Nutrition per taco (based on 10 servings):

- Calories: 150
- Total Fat: 8g
- Saturated Fat: 2g
- Cholesterol: 5mg
- Sodium: 250mg
- Total Carbohydrates: 16g
- Fiber: 4g
- Sugars: 2g
- Protein: 5g

2.11 Grilled Veggie and Hummus Wrap

Ingredients:

- 1 zucchini, sliced lengthwise into 1/4-inch thick strips
- 1 red bell pepper, sliced into strips
- 1 yellow squash, sliced lengthwise into 1/4-inch thick strips
- 1 red onion, sliced into 1/2-inch thick rounds
- 2 tablespoons olive oil
- Salt and pepper to taste
- 1/2 cup your favorite hummus (such as roasted red pepper, garlic, or tomato basil)
- 4 large whole wheat or spinach tortillas
- 2 cups baby spinach or arugula

Instructions:

1. Preheat a grill or grill pan to medium-high heat.
2. In a large bowl, toss the zucchini, bell pepper, yellow squash, and red onion slices with the olive oil. Season with salt and pepper.
3. Grill the vegetables for 2-3 minutes per side, until tender and lightly charred. Transfer the grilled veggies to a plate.
4. Spread about 2 tablespoons of hummus onto the center of each tortilla, leaving a 1-inch border.
5. Top the hummus with a portion of the grilled vegetables and a handful of baby spinach or arugula.
6. Fold the bottom of the tortilla up over the filling, then fold in the sides and continue rolling tightly into a wrap.
7. Serve the grilled veggie and hummus wraps immediately.

Cooking Time:

- Prep Time: 15 minutes

- Cook Time: 10 minutes
- Total Time: 25 minutes

Serving and Nutrition:

This recipe makes 4 wraps, with 1 wrap per serving.

Nutrition per serving:

- Calories: 350
- Total Fat: 16g
- Saturated Fat: 2g
- Cholesterol: 0mg
- Sodium: 550mg
- Total Carbohydrates: 45g
- Fiber: 8g
- Sugars: 5g
- Protein: 10g

2.12 Lemon Garlic Shrimp Salad

Ingredients:

For the Shrimp:

- 1 pound large shrimp, peeled and deveined
- 2 tablespoons olive oil
- 1 tablespoon lemon juice
- 1 teaspoon garlic powder
- Salt and pepper to taste

For the Shrimp:

- 1 pound large shrimp, peeled and deveined
- 2 tablespoons olive oil
- 1 tablespoon lemon juice
- 1 teaspoon garlic powder
- Salt and pepper to taste

For the Salad:

- 1 head of romaine lettuce, chopped
- 1 cup cherry tomatoes, halved
- 1/2 cup crumbled feta cheese
- 1/4 cup chopped fresh parsley
- 1/4 cup chopped fresh dill
- 2 tablespoons chopped fresh chives

For the Dressing:

- 1/4 cup olive oil
- 2 tablespoons lemon juice
- 1 tablespoon Dijon mustard
- 1 teaspoon garlic powder

- Salt and pepper to taste

Instructions:

1. **Marinate the Shrimp:** In a large bowl, toss the shrimp with the olive oil, lemon juice, garlic powder, salt, and pepper. Cover and refrigerate for at least 30 minutes to 1 hour.
2. **Cook the Shrimp:** Preheat a grill or grill pan to medium-high heat. Grill the shrimp for 2-3 minutes per side, until cooked through. Remove from heat and let cool slightly.
3. **Prepare the Salad:** In a large bowl, combine the chopped romaine lettuce, halved cherry tomatoes, crumbled feta cheese, chopped parsley, chopped dill, and chopped chives.
4. **Make the Dressing:** In a small bowl, whisk together the olive oil, lemon juice, Dijon mustard, garlic powder, salt, and pepper.
5. **Assemble the Salad:** Add the cooked shrimp to the salad bowl. Drizzle the dressing over the salad and toss gently to coat everything evenly.
6. **Serve:** Serve the lemon garlic shrimp salad immediately.

Cooking Time:

- **Marinating Time:** 30 minutes to 1 hour
- **Cooking Time:** 4-6 minutes
- **Total Time:** 34-66 minutes

Serving and Nutrition:

This recipe makes 4-6 servings, depending on portion size.

Nutrition per serving (based on 6 servings):

- Calories: 250
- Total Fat: 14g
- Saturated Fat: 3g
- Cholesterol: 120mg
- Sodium: 320mg
- Total Carbohydrates: 20g

- Fiber: 4g
- Sugars: 5g
- Protein: 20g

2.13 Rainbow Veggie Bowl

Ingredients:

- 1 cup cooked quinoa
- 1 cup shredded purple cabbage
- 1 cup shredded carrots
- 1 cup diced cucumber
- 1 cup cherry tomatoes, halved
- 1/2 cup diced avocado
- 2 tablespoons toasted pumpkin seeds
- 2 tablespoons crumbled feta cheese (optional)
- 2 tablespoons balsamic vinaigrette (or dressing of your choice)

Instructions:

1. Cook the quinoa according to package instructions. Allow to cool slightly.
2. In a large bowl, combine the cooked quinoa, shredded purple cabbage, shredded carrots, diced cucumber, halved cherry tomatoes, and diced avocado.
3. Top the veggie bowl with the toasted pumpkin seeds and crumbled feta cheese (if using).
4. Drizzle the balsamic vinaigrette (or dressing of your choice) over the top.
5. Gently toss the ingredients together until everything is evenly coated with the dressing.
6. Serve the Rainbow Veggie Bowl immediately, or refrigerate until ready to enjoy.

Cooking Time:

- Prep Time: 15 minutes
- Cook Time: 15-20 minutes (for quinoa)
- Total Time: 30-35 minutes

Serving and Nutrition:

This recipe makes 2 large servings or 4 smaller servings.

Nutrition per large serving (without feta):

- Calories: 350
- Total Fat: 16g
- Saturated Fat: 2g
- Cholesterol: 0mg
- Sodium: 120mg
- Total Carbohydrates: 44g
- Fiber: 10g
- Sugars: 10g
- Protein: 12g

2.14 Stuffed Bell Peppers with Quinoa

Ingredients:

- 4 bell peppers (any color), halved lengthwise and seeds removed
- 1 cup cooked quinoa
- 1 cup diced tomatoes
- 1/2 cup diced onion
- 1/2 cup diced zucchini
- 1/4 cup crumbled feta cheese
- 2 tablespoons chopped fresh basil
- 1 tablespoon olive oil
- 1 teaspoon dried oregano
- Salt and black pepper to taste

Instructions:

1. Preheat the oven to 375°F (190°C).
2. Place the bell pepper halves cut-side up in a baking dish. Lightly spray or brush with olive oil and season with salt and pepper. Bake for 15 minutes to partially cook the peppers.
3. In a medium bowl, combine the cooked quinoa, diced tomatoes, onion, zucchini, feta cheese, basil, olive oil, oregano, salt, and black pepper. Mix well.
4. Spoon the quinoa mixture evenly into the partially baked bell pepper halves.
5. Cover the baking dish with foil and bake for an additional 20-25 minutes, or until the peppers are tender and the filling is hot.
6. Remove the foil during the last 5 minutes of baking to allow the tops to brown slightly.
7. Serve the stuffed bell peppers warm.

Cooking Time:

- Prep Time: 15 minutes

- Cook Time: 40-45 minutes
- Total Time: 55-60 minutes

Serving and Nutrition:

This recipe makes 8 stuffed bell pepper halves, with 1 half per serving.

Nutrition per serving:

- Calories: 120
- Total Fat: 4g
- Saturated Fat: 1g
- Cholesterol: 5mg
- Sodium: 210mg
- Total Carbohydrates: 16g
- Fiber: 3g
- Sugars: 5g
- Protein: 6g

2.15 Spinach and Berry Salad

Ingredients:

For the Salad:

- 6 cups baby spinach
- 1 cup strawberries, halved
- 1/2 cup raspberries
- 1/2 cup blueberries
- 1/3 cup goat cheese, crumbled
- 1/3 cup red onion, thinly sliced
- 1/4 cup pecans, roughly chopped

For the Dressing:

- 1/2 recipe Raspberry Vinaigrette

Instructions:

1. **Prepare the Salad:** In a large bowl, combine the baby spinach, halved strawberries, raspberries, blueberries, crumbled goat cheese, thinly sliced red onion, and roughly chopped pecans.
2. **Add the Dressing:** Drizzle the Raspberry Vinaigrette over the salad and toss gently to coat everything evenly.
3. **Serve:** Serve the spinach and berry salad immediately.

Cooking Time:

- **Prep Time:** 10 minutes
- **Total Time:** 10 minutes

Serving and Nutrition:

This recipe makes 4-6 servings, depending on portion size.

Nutrition per serving (based on 6 servings):

- **Calories:** 283

- **Total Fat:** 20.6g
- **Saturated Fat:** 6g
- **Cholesterol:** 13.7mg
- **Sodium:** 295mg
- **Total Carbohydrates:** 16.7g
- **Fiber:** 7.2g
- **Sugars:** 6.2g
- **Protein:** 10.2g

Chapter:3 Snack Recipes

3.1 Hummus and Veggie Platter

Ingredients:

- 1 cup hummus (any flavor of your choice, such as classic, roasted red pepper, or basil pesto)
- 1 cup baby carrots
- 1 cup cucumber slices
- 1 cup cherry tomatoes, halved
- 1 cup broccoli florets
- 1 cup cauliflower florets
- 1 cup bell pepper strips (any color)
- 1 cup snap peas or snow peas
- 1 cup whole grain pita chips or crackers

Instructions:

1. Arrange the hummus in the center of a large platter or board.
2. Surround the hummus with the prepared vegetables, grouping them by color or type for a visually appealing presentation.
3. Place the pita chips or crackers around the edges of the platter.
4. Serve immediately, allowing guests to scoop up the hummus and dip the vegetables and pita chips as desired.

Cooking Time:

- Prep Time: 15 minutes
- Total Time: 15 minutes

Serving and Nutrition:

This platter makes a great appetizer or snack for 4-6 people, depending on portion sizes.

Nutrition per serving (based on 6 servings):

- Calories: 200
- Total Fat: 10g
- Saturated Fat: 1.5g
- Cholesterol: 0mg
- Sodium: 400mg
- Total Carbohydrates: 25g
- Fiber: 7g
- Sugars: 5g
- Protein: 7g

3.2 Fresh Fruit Salad

Ingredients:

- 1 cup diced pineapple
- 1 cup diced mango
- 1 cup halved strawberries
- 1 cup blueberries
- 1 cup diced kiwi
- 2 tablespoons fresh lime juice
- 1 tablespoon honey
- 1/4 cup chopped fresh mint leaves

Instructions:

1. In a large bowl, combine the diced pineapple, mango, strawberries, blueberries, and kiwi.
2. In a small bowl, whisk together the lime juice and honey to make the dressing.
3. Pour the dressing over the fruit and gently toss to coat evenly.
4. Sprinkle the chopped fresh mint leaves over the top of the fruit salad.
5. Serve immediately or refrigerate until ready to serve.

Cooking Time:

- Prep Time: 15 minutes
- Total Time: 15 minutes

Serving and Nutrition:

This recipe makes 4 servings. Each serving contains:

- Calories: 135
- Total Fat: 1g
- Saturated Fat: 0g
- Cholesterol: 0mg

- Sodium: 2mg
- Total Carbohydrates: 34g
- Fiber: 5g
- Sugars: 27g
- Protein: 2g

3.3 Roasted Chickpeas

Ingredients:

- 1 (15 oz) can chickpeas, drained and rinsed
- 1 tablespoon olive oil
- 1 teaspoon ground cumin
- 1/2 teaspoon chili powder
- 1/4 teaspoon garlic powder
- 1/4 teaspoon salt

Instructions:

1. Preheat the oven to 400°F (200°C). Line a baking sheet with parchment paper.
2. Pat the drained and rinsed chickpeas dry with paper towels or a clean kitchen towel. Remove any loose skins.
3. In a medium bowl, toss the chickpeas with olive oil, cumin, chili powder, garlic powder, and salt until evenly coated.
4. Spread the chickpeas in a single layer on the prepared baking sheet.
5. Roast for 20-25 minutes, shaking the pan halfway, until the chickpeas are crispy and golden brown.
6. Remove from the oven and let cool for 5 minutes before serving.

Cooking Time:

- Prep Time: 5 minutes
- Cook Time: 20-25 minutes
- Total Time: 25-30 minutes

Serving and Nutrition:

This recipe makes about 1 cup of roasted chickpeas, which can be divided into 2-4 servings depending on how they are used.

Nutrition per 1/2 cup serving:

- Calories: 150
- Total Fat: 5g
- Saturated Fat: 1g
- Cholesterol: 0mg
- Sodium: 360mg
- Total Carbohydrates: 20g
- Fiber: 5g
- Sugars: 2g
- Protein: 6g

3.4 Greek Yogurt with Honey and Walnuts

Ingredients:

- 4 cups (960g) full-fat Greek yogurt
- 1/2 cup (120ml) honey
- 1 cup (120g) chopped toasted walnuts

Instructions:

1. Toast the walnuts: In a dry skillet over medium heat, toast the walnuts for 5-7 minutes, stirring frequently, until fragrant and lightly browned. Allow to cool completely.
2. In a large bowl, stir the Greek yogurt until smooth and creamy.
3. Divide the yogurt evenly between 4-6 serving bowls or glasses.
4. Drizzle 2-3 tablespoons of honey over the top of each serving of yogurt.
5. Sprinkle the toasted chopped walnuts over the honey-drizzled yogurt.
6. Serve immediately and enjoy!

Cooking Time:

- Prep Time: 10 minutes
- Cook Time: 5-7 minutes (for toasting walnuts)
- Total Time: 15-17 minutes

Serving and Nutrition:

This recipe makes 4-6 servings, depending on portion size.

Nutrition per serving (based on 4 servings):

- Calories: 390
- Total Fat: 20g
- Saturated Fat: 5g
- Cholesterol: 35mg
- Sodium: 115mg
- Total Carbohydrates: 35g

- Fiber: 3g
- Sugars: 30g
- Protein: 20g

3.5 Cucumber and Tomato Salad

Ingredients:

- 3 cups diced cucumber (about 1 large or 2 medium cucumbers)
- 2 cups halved cherry or grape tomatoes
- 1/2 cup thinly sliced red onion
- 2 tablespoons chopped fresh basil
- 2 tablespoons olive oil
- 1 tablespoon red wine vinegar
- 1 teaspoon Dijon mustard
- 1/2 teaspoon salt
- 1/4 teaspoon black pepper

Instructions:

1. In a large bowl, combine the diced cucumber, halved tomatoes, sliced red onion, and chopped basil.
2. In a small bowl, whisk together the olive oil, red wine vinegar, Dijon mustard, salt, and black pepper to make the dressing.
3. Pour the dressing over the cucumber and tomato mixture and toss gently to coat.
4. Cover and refrigerate for at least 30 minutes to allow the flavors to meld.
5. Serve chilled or at room temperature.

Cooking Time:

- Prep Time: 15 minutes
- Chilling Time: 30 minutes
- Total Time: 45 minutes

Serving and Nutrition:

This recipe makes 4-6 servings, depending on portion size.

Nutrition per serving (based on 6 servings):

- Calories: 90

- Total Fat: 6g
- Saturated Fat: 1g
- Cholesterol: 0mg
- Sodium: 290mg
- Total Carbohydrates: 8g
- Fiber: 2g
- Sugars: 4g
- Protein: 2g

3.6 Bell Pepper Strips with Guacamole

Ingredients:

For the Bell Pepper Strips:

- 2 large bell peppers (any color), sliced into 1/2-inch thick strips
- 1 tablespoon olive oil
- 1/4 teaspoon salt
- 1/4 teaspoon black pepper

For the Guacamole:

- 2 ripe avocados, pitted and diced
- 1/4 cup diced red onion
- 2 tablespoons chopped fresh cilantro
- 1 tablespoon lime juice
- 1 garlic clove, minced
- 1/4 teaspoon salt
- 1/4 teaspoon ground cumin

Instructions:

1. **Prepare the Bell Pepper Strips:** Preheat your oven to 400°F (200°C). Line a baking sheet with parchment paper.
2. In a medium bowl, toss the bell pepper strips with the olive oil, salt, and black pepper until evenly coated.
3. Spread the seasoned bell pepper strips in a single layer on the prepared baking sheet.
4. Roast the bell pepper strips for 12-15 minutes, flipping halfway, until they are tender and slightly charred on the edges.
5. **Make the Guacamole:** In a medium bowl, gently mix together the diced avocado, red onion, cilantro, lime juice, garlic, salt, and cumin until well combined.

6. **Serve:** Arrange the roasted bell pepper strips on a serving platter. Serve the guacamole alongside the bell pepper strips for dipping.

Cooking Time:

- Prep Time: 15 minutes
- Cook Time: 12-15 minutes
- Total Time: 27-30 minutes

Serving and Nutrition:

This recipe makes 4-6 servings, depending on portion size.

Nutrition per serving (based on 6 servings):

- Calories: 120
- Total Fat: 9g
- Saturated Fat: 1.5g
- Cholesterol: 0mg
- Sodium: 210mg
- Total Carbohydrates: 10g
- Fiber: 5g
- Sugars: 3g
- Protein: 2g

3.7 Spicy Edamame

Ingredients:

- 1 pound frozen edamame, shelled
- 1/4 cup soy sauce
- 2 tablespoons sesame oil
- 2 cloves garlic, minced
- 1 tablespoon grated fresh ginger
- 1/2 teaspoon red pepper flakes
- 1/4 teaspoon salt
- 1/4 teaspoon black pepper
- 1 tablespoon sesame seeds

Instructions:

1. **Cook the Edamame:** In a large pot, bring 4 cups of water to a boil. Add the frozen edamame and cook for 3-4 minutes, until tender. Drain and set aside.
2. **Make the Spicy Sauce:** In a small bowl, whisk together the soy sauce, sesame oil, minced garlic, grated fresh ginger, red pepper flakes, salt, and black pepper.
3. **Combine and Serve:** Toss the cooked edamame with the spicy sauce until evenly coated.
4. **Sprinkle with Sesame Seeds:** Sprinkle the sesame seeds over the edamame.
5. Serve immediately.

Cooking Time:

- **Cooking Time:** 3-4 minutes
- **Total Time:** 5-6 minutes

Serving and Nutrition:

This recipe makes 4-6 servings, depending on portion size.

Nutrition per serving (based on 6 servings):

- Calories: 120
- Total Fat: 6g
- Saturated Fat: 1g
- Cholesterol: 0mg
- Sodium: 500mg
- Total Carbohydrates: 10g
- Fiber: 4g
- Sugars: 2g
- Protein: 10g

3.8 Apple Slices with Cinnamon

Ingredients:

- 2 medium apples, cored and sliced into 1/4-inch thick wedges
- 1 teaspoon ground cinnamon

Instructions:

1. Wash and core the apples. Slice them into 1/4-inch thick wedges.
2. Arrange the apple slices in a single layer on a plate or baking sheet.
3. Sprinkle the ground cinnamon evenly over the apple slices, making sure to coat both sides.
4. Serve immediately or refrigerate until ready to enjoy.

Cooking Time:

- Prep Time: 5 minutes
- Total Time: 5 minutes

Serving and Nutrition:

This recipe makes 2-3 servings, depending on the size of the apples and how many slices each person enjoys.

Nutrition per serving (based on 3 servings):

- Calories: 80
- Total Fat: 0g
- Saturated Fat: 0g
- Cholesterol: 0mg
- Sodium: 0mg
- Total Carbohydrates: 21g
- Fiber: 4g
- Sugars: 16g
- Protein: 0g

3.9 Mixed Berry Medley

Ingredients:

- 1 cup fresh strawberries, hulled and halved
- 1 cup fresh blueberries
- 1 cup fresh raspberries
- 1 cup fresh blackberries
- 2 tablespoons honey (or maple syrup)
- 1 tablespoon fresh lemon juice

Instructions:

1. In a large bowl, gently combine the strawberries, blueberries, raspberries, and blackberries.
2. Drizzle the honey (or maple syrup) and lemon juice over the berries, and gently toss to coat.
3. Cover and refrigerate the mixed berry medley for at least 30 minutes, or up to 4 hours, to allow the flavors to meld.
4. Serve the berry medley chilled, either on its own as a snack or as a topping for yogurt, oatmeal, pancakes, waffles, or other desserts.

Cooking Time:

- Prep Time: 10 minutes
- Chilling Time: 30 minutes to 4 hours
- Total Time: 40 minutes to 4 hours 10 minutes

Serving and Nutrition:

This recipe makes approximately 4 cups of mixed berry medley, which can serve 4-6 people as a snack or topping.

Nutrition per 1/2 cup serving:

- Calories: 80
- Total Fat: 1g

- Saturated Fat: 0g
- Cholesterol: 0mg
- Sodium: 0mg
- Total Carbohydrates: 18g
- Fiber: 4g
- Sugars: 12g
- Protein: 1g

3.10 Carrot and Celery Sticks with Hummus

Ingredients:

For the Sticks:

- 6 medium carrots, peeled and cut into sticks
- 6 medium celery stalks, cut into sticks

For the Hummus:

- 1 cup hummus (any flavor of your choice)

Instructions:

1. **Prepare the Sticks:** Wash and cut the carrots and celery into sticks. Pat them dry with paper towels or a clean kitchen towel.
2. **Make the Hummus:** If using store-bought hummus, simply scoop it into a serving bowl. If making your own hummus, follow your favorite recipe.
3. **Assemble:** Place the carrot and celery sticks on a serving platter or in a snack bowl.
4. **Serve:** Serve the carrot and celery sticks with the hummus for dipping.

Cooking Time:

- **Prep Time:** 10 minutes
- **Total Time:** 10 minutes

Serving and Nutrition:

This recipe makes 6 servings, depending on the size of the sticks and how many are eaten per serving.

Nutrition per serving (based on 6 servings):

- **Calories:** 120
- **Total Fat:** 6g
- **Saturated Fat:** 1g
- **Cholesterol:** 0mg

- **Sodium:** 120mg
- **Total Carbohydrates:** 15g
- **Fiber:** 5g
- **Sugars:** 5g
- **Protein:** 5g

3.11 Watermelon Cubes with Mint

Ingredients:

- 4 cups cubed watermelon (about 1/2 a medium watermelon)
- 1/4 cup chopped fresh mint leaves
- 1 tablespoon lime juice
- 1/4 teaspoon salt

Instructions:

1. In a large bowl, combine the cubed watermelon, chopped mint leaves, lime juice, and salt. Gently toss to mix everything together.
2. Serve the watermelon cubes with mint immediately, or refrigerate for up to 2 hours before serving to allow the flavors to meld.

Cooking Time:

- Prep Time: 10 minutes
- Total Time: 10 minutes

Serving and Nutrition:

This recipe makes 4 servings.

Nutrition per serving:

- Calories: 70
- Total Fat: 0g
- Saturated Fat: 0g
- Cholesterol: 0mg
- Sodium: 120mg
- Total Carbohydrates: 18g
- Fiber: 1g
- Sugars: 16g
- Protein: 1g

3.12 Hard-Boiled Eggs

Ingredients:

- Eggs

Instructions:

1. Place the eggs in a single layer in a saucepan and cover with cold water by 1 inch.
2. Bring the water to a boil over high heat.
3. Once the water reaches a full boil, remove the pan from the heat, cover, and let sit for:
    - ❖ **Soft-boiled:** 2-3 minutes
    - ❖ **Hard-boiled:** 10-12 minutes
4. Drain the hot water and cover the eggs with cold water to cool.
5. Once cooled, gently tap each egg on the counter to crack the shell. Peel starting from the wider end of the egg.
6. Rinse the peeled eggs under cold water to remove any shell fragments.
7. Enjoy the hard-boiled eggs as is, or use them in your desired recipe.

Cooking Time:

- **Prep Time:** 5 minutes
- **Cook Time:** 10-12 minutes
- **Total Time:** 15-17 minutes

Serving and Nutrition:

This recipe yields as many hard-boiled eggs as you prepare.

Nutrition per large egg:

- **Calories:** 78
- **Total Fat:** 5g
- **Saturated Fat:** 2g
- **Cholesterol:** 186mg
- **Sodium:** 62mg

- **Total Carbohydrates:** 0g
- **Fiber:** 0g
- **Sugars:** 0g
- **Protein:** 6g

3.13 Kale Chips

Ingredients:

- 1 bunch of kale, washed and dried thoroughly
- 1-2 tablespoons olive oil or avocado oil
- 1/2 teaspoon salt (or more to taste)
- Optional seasonings: garlic powder, onion powder, chili powder, parmesan cheese, etc.

Instructions:

1. Preheat your oven to 325°F (165°C).
2. Wash the kale and thoroughly dry it using a salad spinner or paper towels. This is crucial for getting crispy kale chips.
3. Remove the tough stems from the kale leaves and tear or cut the leaves into bite-sized pieces.
4. In a large bowl, toss the kale leaves with the olive oil and salt until the leaves are evenly coated.
5. Spread the kale leaves in a single layer on one or two large baking sheets, making sure they don't overlap.
6. Bake for 12-18 minutes, flipping the leaves halfway through, until the kale is crispy and lightly browned on the edges.
7. Remove the kale chips from the oven and let them cool for a few minutes. They will continue to crisp up as they cool.
8. Optionally, you can sprinkle on any additional seasonings like garlic powder, onion powder, chili powder, or parmesan cheese.
9. Serve the kale chips immediately for maximum crispness.

Cooking and Prep Time:

- Prep Time: 10-15 minutes
- Cook Time: 12-18 minutes

- Total Time: 22-33 minutes

Serving and Nutrition:

This recipe makes approximately 4 servings of kale chips.

Nutrition per serving (based on 4 servings):

- Calories: 60
- Total Fat: 4g
- Saturated Fat: 0.5g
- Cholesterol: 0mg
- Sodium: 230mg
- Total Carbohydrates: 5g
- Fiber: 1g
- Sugars: 0g
- Protein: 2g

3.14 Salsa with Cucumber Rounds

Ingredients:

For the Salsa:

- 2 cups diced tomatoes (about 3-4 medium tomatoes)
- 1/2 cup diced red onion
- 1/4 cup chopped fresh cilantro
- 2 tablespoons lime juice
- 1 jalapeño, seeded and finely chopped (optional, for spice)
- 1 garlic clove, minced
- 1/2 teaspoon salt
- 1/4 teaspoon black pepper

For the Cucumber Rounds:

- 2 medium cucumbers, sliced into 1/4-inch thick rounds

Instructions:

1. **Make the Salsa:** In a medium bowl, combine the diced tomatoes, red onion, cilantro, lime juice, jalapeño (if using), garlic, salt, and black pepper. Stir to mix well.
2. **Prepare the Cucumber Rounds:** Slice the cucumbers into 1/4-inch thick rounds.
3. **Assemble:** Place a spoonful of the salsa on top of each cucumber round.
4. **Serve:** Serve the salsa-topped cucumber rounds immediately, or refrigerate until ready to serve.

Cooking and Prep Time:

- Prep Time: 15 minutes
- Total Time: 15 minutes

Serving and Nutrition:

This recipe makes approximately 16-20 salsa-topped cucumber rounds, depending on the size of the cucumbers.

Nutrition per 2 cucumber rounds with salsa (based on 20 servings):

- Calories: 25
- Total Fat: 0g
- Saturated Fat: 0g
- Cholesterol: 0mg
- Sodium: 105mg
- Total Carbohydrates: 6g
- Fiber: 1g
- Sugars: 3g
- Protein: 1g

3.15 Berry and Yogurt Parfait

Ingredients:

- 2 cups plain Greek yogurt
- 1 cup mixed fresh berries (such as raspberries, blueberries, and strawberries)
- 1/2 cup granola
- 2 tablespoons honey (optional)

Instructions:

1. In a parfait glass or small bowl, layer 1/4 cup of yogurt.
2. Top the yogurt with 1/4 cup of mixed berries.
3. Sprinkle 2 tablespoons of granola over the berries.
4. Repeat the layers of yogurt, berries, and granola two more times, ending with a layer of granola.
5. If desired, drizzle 1 tablespoon of honey over the top of the parfait.
6. Refrigerate the parfait until ready to serve.

Cooking and Prep Time:

- Prep Time: 10 minutes
- Total Time: 10 minutes

Serving and Nutrition:

This recipe makes 2 servings of berry and yogurt parfait.

Nutrition per serving:

- Calories: 300
- Total Fat: 5g
- Saturated Fat: 1g
- Cholesterol: 15mg
- Sodium: 105mg
- Total Carbohydrates: 45g
- Fiber: 5g

- Sugars: 30g
- Protein: 20g

Chapter:4 Dinner Recipes

4.1 Baked Salmon with Asparagus

Ingredients:

- 1 lb salmon fillets, cut into 4 portions
- 1 lb asparagus spears, trimmed
- 2 tablespoons olive oil
- 1 teaspoon garlic powder
- 1 teaspoon dried dill
- 1/2 teaspoon salt
- 1/4 teaspoon black pepper
- 1 lemon, cut into wedges (for serving)

Instructions:

1. Preheat your oven to 400°F (200°C). Line a large baking sheet with parchment paper or foil.
2. Place the salmon fillets and asparagus spears on the prepared baking sheet. Drizzle with the olive oil and sprinkle with the garlic powder, dried dill, salt, and black pepper. Toss to coat everything evenly.
3. Arrange the salmon and asparagus in a single layer on the baking sheet, making sure they are not overlapping.
4. Bake for 12-15 minutes, or until the salmon is cooked through and flakes easily with a fork, and the asparagus is tender-crisp.
5. Serve the baked salmon and asparagus immediately, with lemon wedges on the side.

Cooking and Prep Time:

- Prep Time: 10 minutes
- Cook Time: 12-15 minutes

- Total Time: 22-25 minutes

Serving and Nutrition:

This recipe makes 4 servings.

Nutrition per serving:

- Calories: 300
- Total Fat: 16g
- Saturated Fat: 3g
- Cholesterol: 80mg
- Sodium: 420mg
- Total Carbohydrates: 8g
- Fiber: 3g
- Sugars: 3g
- Protein: 32g

4.2 Turkey and Veggie Stuffed Peppers

Ingredients:

- 6 bell peppers (any color), halved lengthwise and seeds removed
- 1 lb ground turkey
- 1 cup diced onion
- 1 cup diced zucchini
- 1 cup diced tomatoes
- 1/2 cup cooked brown rice
- 2 cloves garlic, minced
- 1 teaspoon dried oregano
- 1/2 teaspoon ground cumin
- 1/4 teaspoon red pepper flakes (optional)
- Salt and black pepper to taste
- 1/2 cup shredded mozzarella cheese (optional)

Instructions:

1. Preheat your oven to 375°F (190°C).
2. In a large skillet over medium heat, cook the ground turkey, breaking it up as it cooks, until no longer pink, about 5-7 minutes.
3. Add the diced onion, zucchini, and tomatoes to the skillet. Cook for an additional 5 minutes, stirring occasionally, until the vegetables are tender.
4. Stir in the cooked brown rice, garlic, oregano, cumin, and red pepper flakes (if using). Season with salt and black pepper to taste.
5. Arrange the bell pepper halves in a baking dish. Spoon the turkey and veggie mixture evenly into the pepper halves.
6. If using, sprinkle the shredded mozzarella cheese over the top of the stuffed peppers.
7. Bake for 25-30 minutes, or until the peppers are tender and the filling is hot.
8. Serve the turkey and veggie stuffed peppers warm.

Cooking and Prep Time:

- Prep Time: 20 minutes
- Cook Time: 30-35 minutes
- Total Time: 50-55 minutes

Serving and Nutrition:

This recipe makes 6 servings, with 1 stuffed pepper half per serving.

Nutrition per serving:

- Calories: 250
- Total Fat: 10g
- Saturated Fat: 3g
- Cholesterol: 65mg
- Sodium: 320mg
- Total Carbohydrates: 20g
- Fiber: 5g
- Sugars: 7g
- Protein: 22g

4.3 Spaghetti Squash with Marinara Sauce

Ingredients:

- 1 medium spaghetti squash, halved lengthwise and seeds removed
- 1 tablespoon olive oil
- Salt and black pepper to taste
- 1 batch of Marinara Sauce (see recipe below)

For the Marinara Sauce:

- 2 tablespoons olive oil
- 1 onion, diced
- 3 cloves garlic, minced
- 1 (28 oz) can crushed tomatoes
- 2 tablespoons tomato paste
- 1 teaspoon dried oregano
- 1/2 teaspoon dried basil
- 1/4 teaspoon red pepper flakes (optional)
- Salt and black pepper to taste

Instructions:

For the Spaghetti Squash:

1. Preheat the oven to 400°F (200°C).
2. Place the spaghetti squash halves cut-side up on a baking sheet. Drizzle with olive oil and season with salt and pepper.
3. Roast for 40-50 minutes, until the squash is tender and can be easily shredded with a fork.
4. Let the squash cool slightly, then use a fork to shred the flesh into spaghetti-like strands.

For the Marinara Sauce:

1. In a large saucepan, heat the olive oil over medium heat. Add the diced onion and sauté for 5-7 minutes until translucent.
2. Add the minced garlic and cook for 1 minute until fragrant.
3. Stir in the crushed tomatoes, tomato paste, oregano, basil, and red pepper flakes (if using). Season with salt and pepper to taste.
4. Bring the sauce to a simmer and let it cook for 15-20 minutes, stirring occasionally, until thickened.

Assemble the Dish:

1. Toss the roasted spaghetti squash strands with the marinara sauce until well coated.
2. Serve hot, garnished with additional fresh basil or parmesan cheese if desired.

Cooking and Prep Time:

- Prep Time: 15 minutes
- Cook Time: 55-65 minutes (40-50 minutes for squash, 15-20 minutes for sauce)
- Total Time: 70-80 minutes

Serving and Nutrition:

This recipe makes 4 servings.

Nutrition per serving:

- Calories: 220
- Total Fat: 9g
- Saturated Fat: 1g
- Cholesterol: 0mg
- Sodium: 590mg
- Total Carbohydrates: 32g
- Fiber: 7g

- Sugars: 12g
- Protein: 5g

4.4 Grilled Portobello Mushrooms

Ingredients:

- 4 large portobello mushroom caps, stems removed
- 2 tablespoons olive oil
- 2 tablespoons balsamic vinegar
- 2 cloves garlic, minced
- 1 teaspoon dried thyme
- 1/2 teaspoon salt
- 1/4 teaspoon black pepper

Instructions:

1. In a shallow baking dish or resealable plastic bag, combine the olive oil, balsamic vinegar, garlic, thyme, salt, and pepper. Add the portobello mushroom caps and toss to coat them evenly with the marinade.
2. Cover the dish or seal the bag and let the mushrooms marinate for 30 minutes to 1 hour, flipping them occasionally.
3. Preheat your grill or grill pan to medium-high heat.
4. Grill the marinated portobello mushrooms for 4-5 minutes per side, or until they are tender and have grill marks.
5. Serve the grilled portobello mushrooms immediately, either as a main dish or as a side. They pair well with grilled vegetables, salads, or grain bowls.

Cooking and Prep Time:

- Prep Time: 10 minutes
- Marinating Time: 30 minutes to 1 hour
- Cook Time: 8-10 minutes
- Total Time: 50 minutes to 1 hour 20 minutes

Serving and Nutrition:

This recipe makes 4 servings, with 1 portobello mushroom cap per serving.

Nutrition per serving:

- Calories: 110
- Total Fat: 8g
- Saturated Fat: 1g
- Cholesterol: 0mg
- Sodium: 360mg
- Total Carbohydrates: 9g
- Fiber: 2g
- Sugars: 4g
- Protein: 3g

4.5 Cauliflower Fried Rice

Ingredients:

- 1 head of cauliflower, cut into florets
- 2 tablespoons olive oil
- 1 onion, diced
- 2 cloves garlic, minced
- 1 cup frozen peas and carrots
- 2 eggs, beaten
- 3 tablespoons soy sauce
- 1 teaspoon sesame oil
- Salt and black pepper to taste
- Chopped green onions for garnish (optional)

Instructions:

1. In a food processor, pulse the cauliflower florets until they resemble rice-sized grains. Set aside.
2. In a large skillet or wok, heat the olive oil over medium-high heat. Add the diced onion and sauté for 2-3 minutes until translucent.
3. Add the minced garlic and sauté for an additional minute until fragrant.
4. Add the riced cauliflower and frozen peas and carrots to the skillet. Stir-fry for 5-7 minutes, until the cauliflower is tender.
5. Push the cauliflower mixture to the side of the skillet. Pour the beaten eggs into the empty side and scramble them, breaking them up into small pieces as they cook.
6. Once the eggs are cooked, mix them into the cauliflower mixture.
7. Add the soy sauce and sesame oil to the skillet. Stir everything together until well combined and heated through.
8. Season with salt and black pepper to taste.

9. Serve the cauliflower fried rice hot, garnished with chopped green onions if
    desired.

Cooking and Prep Time:

- Prep Time: 10 minutes
- Cook Time: 15 minutes
- Total Time: 25 minutes

Serving and Nutrition:

This recipe makes 4 servings.

Nutrition per serving:

- Calories: 150
- Total Fat: 8g
- Saturated Fat: 1g
- Cholesterol: 95mg
- Sodium: 600mg
- Total Carbohydrates: 13g
- Fiber: 4g
- Sugars: 4g
- Protein: 7g

4.6 Lemon Herb Grilled Chicken

Ingredients:

- 4 boneless, skinless chicken breasts
- 1/4 cup olive oil
- 2 tablespoons lemon juice
- 2 tablespoons chopped fresh parsley
- 1 tablespoon chopped fresh thyme
- 1 tablespoon chopped fresh rosemary
- 2 cloves garlic, minced
- 1 teaspoon salt
- 1/2 teaspoon black pepper

Instructions:

1. In a large resealable bag or shallow baking dish, combine the olive oil, lemon juice, parsley, thyme, rosemary, garlic, salt, and pepper. Add the chicken breasts and turn to coat them evenly with the marinade.
2. Cover the dish or seal the bag and refrigerate for 30 minutes to 1 hour, turning the chicken occasionally.
3. Preheat your grill or grill pan to medium-high heat.
4. Remove the chicken from the marinade and discard any remaining marinade.
5. Grill the chicken for 5-7 minutes per side, or until it reaches an internal temperature of 165°F (75°C).
6. Transfer the grilled chicken to a clean plate and let it rest for 5 minutes before serving.

Cooking and Prep Time:

- Prep Time: 10 minutes
- Marinating Time: 30 minutes to 1 hour
- Cook Time: 10-14 minutes

- Total Time: 50 minutes to 1 hour 24 minutes

Serving and Nutrition:

This recipe makes 4 servings, with 1 chicken breast per serving.

Nutrition per serving:

- Calories: 250
- Total Fat: 12g
- Saturated Fat: 2g
- Cholesterol: 90mg
- Sodium: 550mg
- Total Carbohydrates: 2g
- Fiber: 0g
- Sugars: 0g
- Protein: 32g

4.7 Eggplant Parmesan

Ingredients:

- 1 medium eggplant, sliced into 1/2-inch thick rounds
- 1 cup panko breadcrumbs
- 1/2 cup grated Parmesan cheese
- 1 teaspoon dried oregano
- 1/2 teaspoon garlic powder
- 1/4 teaspoon salt
- 2 large eggs, beaten
- 1 cup marinara sauce
- 1 cup shredded mozzarella cheese

Instructions:

1. Preheat your oven to 400°F (200°C). Line a baking sheet with parchment paper.
2. In a shallow bowl, combine the panko breadcrumbs, Parmesan cheese, oregano, garlic powder, and salt.
3. Dip the eggplant slices into the beaten eggs, then coat them in the breadcrumb mixture, pressing gently to help it adhere.
4. Arrange the breaded eggplant slices in a single layer on the prepared baking sheet.
5. Bake for 15-18 minutes, flipping the slices halfway through, until the eggplant is tender and the bread is golden brown.
6. Spread 1/2 cup of the marinara sauce in the bottom of a baking dish. Arrange the baked eggplant slices in a single layer on top of the sauce.
7. Sprinkle the mozzarella cheese evenly over the eggplant.
8. Bake for an additional 10-12 minutes, or until the cheese is melted and bubbly.
9. Serve the eggplant Parmesan hot, with the remaining marinara sauce on the side.

Cooking and Prep Time:

- Prep Time: 10 minutes

- Cook Time: 25-30 minutes
- Total Time: 35-40 minutes

Serving and Nutrition:

This recipe makes 4 servings.

Nutrition per serving:

- Calories: 320
- Total Fat: 14g
- Saturated Fat: 6g
- Cholesterol: 105mg
- Sodium: 780mg
- Total Carbohydrates: 32g
- Fiber: 6g
- Sugars: 7g
- Protein: 18g

4.8 Zucchini Lasagna

Ingredients:

- 3 medium zucchinis, sliced lengthwise into 1/4-inch thick strips
- 1 lb ground beef or Italian sausage
- 1 onion, diced
- 3 cloves garlic, minced
- 1 (28 oz) can crushed tomatoes
- 2 tablespoons tomato paste
- 1 teaspoon dried oregano
- 1/2 teaspoon dried basil
- Salt and black pepper to taste
- 1 (15 oz) container ricotta cheese
- 1 egg
- 1/4 cup grated Parmesan cheese
- 2 cups shredded mozzarella cheese, divided

Instructions:

1. Preheat your oven to 375°F (190°C).
2. In a large skillet over medium heat, cook the ground beef or sausage, onion, and garlic until the meat is browned and the vegetables are tender, about 5-7 minutes. Drain any excess fat.
3. Add the crushed tomatoes, tomato paste, oregano, basil, salt, and pepper to the skillet. Stir to combine and let the sauce simmer for 10 minutes.
4. In a medium bowl, mix together the ricotta cheese, egg, Parmesan cheese, and 1/2 cup of the mozzarella cheese.
5. Spread 1 cup of the meat sauce in the bottom of a 9x13 inch baking dish.
6. Layer half of the zucchini strips over the sauce. Top with half of the ricotta mixture and 1/2 cup of mozzarella cheese. Repeat the layers once more.
7. Top with the remaining meat sauce and mozzarella cheese.

8. Bake for 30-35 minutes, until the zucchini is tender and the cheese is melted and bubbly.

9. Let the lasagna cool for 10 minutes before serving.

Cooking and Prep Time:

- Prep Time: 20 minutes
- Cook Time: 35 minutes
- Total Time: 55 minutes

Serving and Nutrition:

This recipe makes 8 servings.

Nutrition per serving:

- Calories: 350
- Total Fat: 20g
- Saturated Fat: 10g
- Cholesterol: 90mg
- Sodium: 650mg
- Total Carbohydrates: 15g
- Fiber: 3g
- Sugars: 7g
- Protein: 30g

4.9 Chicken and Vegetable Skewers

Ingredients:

- 1 lb boneless, skinless chicken breasts, cut into 1-inch cubes
- 1 red bell pepper, cut into 1-inch pieces
- 1 yellow bell pepper, cut into 1-inch pieces
- 1 red onion, cut into 1-inch pieces
- 8 oz mushrooms, halved
- 2 tablespoons olive oil
- 2 tablespoons lemon juice
- 2 cloves garlic, minced
- 1 teaspoon dried oregano
- 1/2 teaspoon dried thyme
- 1/2 teaspoon salt
- 1/4 teaspoon black pepper

Instructions:

1. In a large resealable bag or bowl, combine the chicken, bell peppers, onion, and mushrooms.
2. In a small bowl, whisk together the olive oil, lemon juice, garlic, oregano, thyme, salt, and black pepper. Pour the marinade over the chicken and vegetables and toss to coat evenly.
3. Cover the bag or bowl and refrigerate for at least 30 minutes, or up to 4 hours, allowing the flavors to meld.
4. Preheat your grill or grill pan to medium-high heat.
5. Thread the marinated chicken and vegetables onto metal or soaked wooden skewers, alternating the ingredients.
6. Grill the skewers for 12-15 minutes, turning occasionally, until the chicken is cooked through and the vegetables are tender.

7. Serve the chicken and vegetable skewers hot, garnished with additional lemon wedges if desired.

Cooking and Prep Time:

- Prep Time: 20 minutes
- Marinating Time: 30 minutes to 4 hours
- Cook Time: 12-15 minutes
- Total Time: 1 hour to 4 hours 35 minutes

Serving and Nutrition:

This recipe makes 4-6 servings, with 2-3 skewers per serving.

Nutrition per serving (based on 6 servings):

- Calories: 220
- Total Fat: 8g
- Saturated Fat: 1g
- Cholesterol: 65mg
- Sodium: 350mg
- Total Carbohydrates: 12g
- Fiber: 3g
- Sugars: 6g
- Protein: 25g

4.10 Shrimp and Vegetable Stir-Fry

Ingredients:

- 1 lb large shrimp, peeled and deveined
- 2 tablespoons vegetable or sesame oil
- 3 cloves garlic, minced
- 1 tablespoon grated fresh ginger
- 1 red bell pepper, sliced
- 1 cup broccoli florets
- 1 cup snow peas or snap peas
- 1 cup sliced mushrooms
- 2 tablespoons low-sodium soy sauce
- 1 tablespoon rice vinegar
- 1 teaspoon sesame oil
- 1/4 teaspoon red pepper flakes (optional)
- Salt and black pepper to taste
- Cooked rice or noodles, for serving (optional)

Instructions:

1. **Prepare the Ingredients:** Peel and devein the shrimp. Mince the garlic and grate the ginger. Slice the bell pepper, prepare the broccoli florets, and slice the mushrooms.
2. **Cook the Shrimp:** In a large skillet or wok, heat the 2 tablespoons of vegetable or sesame oil over high heat. Add the shrimp and cook for 2-3 minutes per side, until opaque and cooked through. Transfer the shrimp to a plate and set aside.
3. **Stir-Fry the Vegetables:** In the same skillet, add the minced garlic and grated ginger. Cook for 1 minute, stirring constantly, until fragrant.
4. **Add the Vegetables:** Add the sliced bell pepper, broccoli florets, snow peas or snap peas, and sliced mushrooms to the skillet. Stir-fry for 4-5 minutes, until the vegetables are crisp-tender.

5. **Make the Sauce:** In a small bowl, whisk together the soy sauce, rice vinegar, 1 teaspoon sesame oil, and red pepper flakes (if using).

6. **Combine and Serve:** Return the cooked shrimp to the skillet with the vegetables. Pour the sauce over the top and toss everything together until well combined and heated through.

7. **Serve:** Serve the shrimp and vegetable stir-fry immediately, over cooked rice or noodles if desired.

Cooking and Prep Time:

- Prep Time: 10 minutes
- Cook Time: 15 minutes
- Total Time: 25 minutes

Serving and Nutrition:

This recipe makes 4 servings.

Nutrition per serving:

- Calories: 250
- Total Fat: 9g
- Saturated Fat: 1g
- Cholesterol: 215mg
- Sodium: 550mg
- Total Carbohydrates: 17g
- Fiber: 4g
- Sugars: 5g
- Protein: 25g

4.11 Lentil and Vegetable Stew

Ingredients:

- 1 tablespoon olive oil
- 1 large onion, diced
- 3 cloves garlic, minced
- 2 carrots, peeled and diced
- 2 celery stalks, diced
- 1 red bell pepper, diced
- 1 cup brown or green lentils, rinsed
- 4 cups vegetable broth
- 1 (14.5 oz) can diced tomatoes
- 2 teaspoons dried thyme
- 1 teaspoon dried oregano
- 1/2 teaspoon smoked paprika
- Salt and black pepper to taste
- 2 cups chopped kale or spinach
- 2 tablespoons chopped fresh parsley

Instructions:

1. In a large pot or Dutch oven, heat the olive oil over medium heat. Add the diced onion and sauté for 5 minutes, until translucent.
2. Add the minced garlic and sauté for 1 minute, until fragrant.
3. Stir in the diced carrots, celery, and bell pepper. Cook for 5-7 minutes, until the vegetables start to soften.
4. Add the rinsed lentils, vegetable broth, diced tomatoes, thyme, oregano, and smoked paprika. Season with salt and black pepper to taste.
5. Bring the stew to a boil, then reduce the heat to low, cover, and simmer for 25-30 minutes, or until the lentils are tender.

6. Stir in the chopped kale or spinach and cook for an additional 5 minutes, until the greens are wilted.

7. Remove from heat and stir in the chopped fresh parsley.

8. Serve the lentil and vegetable stew hot, with crusty bread or over cooked grains if desired.

Cooking and Prep Time:

- Prep Time: 15 minutes
- Cook Time: 35-40 minutes
- Total Time: 50-55 minutes

Serving and Nutrition:

This recipe makes 4-6 servings, depending on portion size.

Nutrition per serving (based on 6 servings):

- Calories: 250
- Total Fat: 5g
- Saturated Fat: 1g
- Cholesterol: 0mg
- Sodium: 600mg
- Total Carbohydrates: 40g
- Fiber: 12g
- Sugars: 8g
- Protein: 15g

4.12 Herb-Crusted Cod

Ingredients:

- 4 cod fillets (about 1.5 lbs total)
- 3 tablespoons cream cheese
- 100g (3.5 oz) fresh breadcrumbs
- Zest and juice of 1 lemon
- 2 tablespoons chopped fresh parsley
- 1 tablespoon chopped fresh thyme
- 1 tablespoon olive oil
- Salt and pepper to taste

Instructions:

1. Preheat your oven to 400°F (200°C).
2. In a small bowl, mix together the cream cheese, breadcrumbs, lemon zest and juice, parsley, and thyme until well combined.
3. Season the cod fillets with salt and pepper on both sides.
4. Place the cod fillets in a baking dish and top each one evenly with the breadcrumb mixture, pressing it down gently to adhere.
5. Drizzle the top of the breadcrumb topping with the olive oil.
6. Bake the herb-crusted cod for 15-18 minutes, or until the fish is opaque and flakes easily with a fork, and the topping is golden brown.
7. Serve the herb-crusted cod immediately, garnished with additional fresh parsley if desired.

Cooking and Prep Time:

- Prep Time: 10 minutes
- Cook Time: 15-18 minutes
- Total Time: 25-28 minutes

Serving and Nutrition:

This recipe makes 4 servings, with 1 cod fillet per serving.

Nutrition per serving:

- Calories: 300
- Total Fat: 12g
- Saturated Fat: 4g
- Cholesterol: 90mg
- Sodium: 450mg
- Total Carbohydrates: 15g
- Fiber: 1g
- Sugars: 1g
- Protein: 35g

4.13 Veggie and Bean Chili

Ingredients:

- 2 tablespoons olive oil
- 1 large onion, diced
- 3 cloves garlic, minced
- 1 red bell pepper, diced
- 1 jalapeño, seeded and minced (optional, for spice)
- 2 tablespoons chili powder
- 1 tablespoon ground cumin
- 1 teaspoon dried oregano
- 1/2 teaspoon smoked paprika
- 1/4 teaspoon cayenne pepper (optional)
- 1 (15 oz) can black beans, drained and rinsed
- 1 (15 oz) can kidney beans, drained and rinsed
- 1 (15 oz) can diced tomatoes
- 1 (6 oz) can tomato paste
- 1 cup vegetable broth
- Salt and black pepper to taste
- Chopped fresh cilantro for garnish (optional)

Instructions:

1. In a large pot or Dutch oven, heat the olive oil over medium heat. Add the diced onion and sauté for 5-7 minutes, until translucent.
2. Add the minced garlic, diced bell pepper, and jalapeño (if using). Cook for an additional 2-3 minutes, until fragrant.
3. Stir in the chili powder, cumin, oregano, smoked paprika, and cayenne pepper (if using). Cook for 1 minute, stirring constantly, to toast the spices.
4. Add the drained and rinsed black beans and kidney beans, the diced tomatoes, tomato paste, and vegetable broth. Stir to combine.

5. Bring the chili to a simmer and let it cook for 20-25 minutes, stirring occasionally, until the flavors have melded and the chili has thickened to your desired consistency.

6. Season the chili with salt and black pepper to taste.

7. Serve the veggie and bean chili hot, garnished with chopped fresh cilantro if desired. Enjoy with cornbread, tortilla chips, or your favorite toppings.

Cooking and Prep Time:

- Prep Time: 15 minutes
- Cook Time: 25-30 minutes
- Total Time: 40-45 minutes

Serving and Nutrition:

This recipe makes 4-6 servings, depending on portion size.

Nutrition per serving (based on 6 servings):

- Calories: 300
- Total Fat: 7g
- Saturated Fat: 1g
- Cholesterol: 0mg
- Sodium: 650mg
- Total Carbohydrates: 47g
- Fiber: 14g
- Sugars: 8g
- Protein: 14g

4.14 Tofu and Vegetable Curry

Ingredients:

- 1 block (14 oz) extra-firm tofu, pressed and cubed
- 2 tablespoons coconut oil
- 1 onion, diced
- 3 cloves garlic, minced
- 1 tablespoon grated fresh ginger
- 2 tablespoons curry powder
- 1 teaspoon ground cumin
- 1 teaspoon ground coriander
- 1/4 teaspoon cayenne pepper (optional, for heat)
- 1 red bell pepper, sliced
- 1 cup cauliflower florets
- 1 cup broccoli florets
- 1 (13.5 oz) can coconut milk
- 1 cup vegetable broth
- 2 tablespoons tomato paste
- 1 tablespoon soy sauce or tamari
- Salt and black pepper to taste
- Chopped fresh cilantro for garnish

Instructions:

1. **Prepare the Tofu:** Press the tofu block between paper towels or a clean kitchen towel to remove excess moisture. Cut the tofu into 1-inch cubes.
2. **Cook the Tofu:** In a large skillet or wok, heat the coconut oil over medium-high heat. Add the tofu cubes and cook, stirring occasionally, until golden brown on all sides, about 5-7 minutes. Transfer the crispy tofu to a plate and set aside.

3. **Make the Curry Sauce:** In the same skillet, add the diced onion and sauté for 3-4 minutes until translucent. Add the minced garlic and grated ginger, and cook for 1 minute until fragrant.

4. **Add the Spices:** Stir in the curry powder, cumin, coriander, and cayenne (if using). Cook for 1-2 minutes, stirring constantly, to toast the spices.

5. **Add the Vegetables:** Add the sliced bell pepper, cauliflower florets, and broccoli florets to the skillet. Sauté for 3-4 minutes, until the vegetables start to soften.

6. **Finish the Curry:** Pour in the coconut milk, vegetable broth, and tomato paste. Stir to combine and bring the mixture to a simmer. Reduce the heat to medium-low and let the curry simmer for 10-15 minutes, until the vegetables are tender.

7. **Finish and Serve:** Stir the soy sauce into the curry and season with salt and black pepper to taste. Gently fold in the reserved crispy tofu.

8. Serve the tofu and vegetable curry hot, garnished with chopped fresh cilantro. Enjoy with steamed rice or naan bread.

Cooking and Prep Time:

- Prep Time: 15 minutes
- Cook Time: 25-30 minutes
- Total Time: 40-45 minutes

Serving and Nutrition:

This recipe makes 4 servings.

Nutrition per serving:

- Calories: 350
- Total Fat: 22g
- Saturated Fat: 14g
- Cholesterol: 0mg
- Sodium: 590mg
- Total Carbohydrates: 26g
- Fiber: 7g

- Sugars: 7g
- Protein: 18g

4.15 Spinach and Tomato Stuffed Chicken Breast

Ingredients:

- 4 boneless, skinless chicken breasts
- 2 cups fresh spinach, chopped
- 1/2 cup sun-dried tomatoes, chopped
- 1/2 cup shredded mozzarella cheese
- 2 cloves garlic, minced
- 1 tablespoon olive oil
- Salt and black pepper to taste

Instructions:

1. Preheat your oven to 400°F (200°C).
2. In a medium bowl, combine the chopped spinach, sun-dried tomatoes, mozzarella cheese, and minced garlic. Season with a pinch of salt and pepper.
3. Using a sharp knife, slice each chicken breast horizontally to create a pocket, being careful not to cut all the way through.
4. Stuff the spinach and tomato mixture evenly into the pockets of the chicken breasts.
5. Heat the olive oil in a large oven-safe skillet or baking dish over medium-high heat.
6. Carefully place the stuffed chicken breasts in the hot skillet or baking dish. Sear the chicken for 2-3 minutes per side to get a nice golden-brown crust.
7. Transfer the skillet or baking dish to the preheated oven and bake for 20-25 minutes, or until the chicken is cooked through and the internal temperature reaches 165°F (75°C).
8. Remove the stuffed chicken breasts from the oven and let them rest for 5 minutes before serving.

Cooking and Prep Time:

- Prep Time: 15 minutes
- Cook Time: 25-30 minutes
- Total Time: 40-45 minutes

Serving and Nutrition:

This recipe makes 4 servings, with 1 stuffed chicken breast per serving.

Nutrition per serving:

- Calories: 300
- Total Fat: 12g
- Saturated Fat: 4g
- Cholesterol: 100mg
- Sodium: 450mg
- Total Carbohydrates: 8g
- Fiber: 2g
- Sugars: 3g
- Protein: 40g

Chapter:5 Side Dish Recipes

5.1 Garlic Roasted Brussels Sprouts

Ingredients:

- 1 pound Brussels sprouts, trimmed and halved
- 2 tablespoons olive oil
- 2 cloves garlic, minced
- Salt and black pepper to taste
- Fresh parsley leaves, for garnish (optional)

Instructions:

1. **Preheat the Oven:** Preheat your oven to 425°F (220°C).
2. **Prepare the Brussels Sprouts:** Trim and halve the Brussels sprouts. Remove any yellow or damaged leaves.
3. **Season and Toss:** In a large bowl, toss the Brussels sprouts with olive oil, minced garlic, salt, and black pepper until they are evenly coated.
4. **Roast:** Transfer the Brussels sprouts to a parchment-lined baking sheet. Arrange them in a single layer with the cut sides facing down.
5. **Bake:** Roast the Brussels sprouts for 20-25 minutes, or until they are tender and lightly charred. Shake the pan halfway through the cooking time to ensure even browning.
6. **Garnish and Serve:** Remove the Brussels sprouts from the oven and garnish with fresh parsley leaves if desired. Serve hot.

Cooking and Prep Time:

- Prep Time: 10 minutes
- Cook Time: 20-25 minutes
- Total Time: 30-35 minutes

Serving and Nutrition:

This recipe makes 4 servings.

Nutrition per serving:

- Calories: 120
- Total Fat: 8g
- Saturated Fat: 1g
- Cholesterol: 0mg
- Sodium: 120mg
- Total Carbohydrates: 12g
- Fiber: 4g
- Sugars: 4g
- Protein: 4g

5.2 Cauliflower Mash

Ingredients:

- 1 large head of cauliflower, cut into florets (about 6 cups)
- 2 tablespoons unsalted butter or olive oil
- 1/4 cup milk, cream, or unsweetened almond milk
- 1/4 cup grated Parmesan cheese (optional)
- 1 clove garlic, minced (optional)
- Salt and black pepper to taste

Instructions:

1. **Prepare the Cauliflower:** Cut the cauliflower into small florets. Place the florets in a large pot and cover with water.
2. **Cook the Cauliflower:** Bring the water to a boil over high heat. Reduce the heat to medium-low and simmer the cauliflower for 10-15 minutes, or until very tender when pierced with a fork.
3. **Drain the Cauliflower:** Drain the cooked cauliflower in a colander and let it cool slightly.
4. **Mash the Cauliflower:** Transfer the drained cauliflower to a food processor or high-powered blender. Add the butter or olive oil, milk, Parmesan cheese (if using), and garlic (if using). Season with salt and black pepper to taste.
5. **Blend until Smooth:** Blend the cauliflower mixture until it reaches a smooth, creamy consistency, scraping down the sides as needed.
6. **Serve and Enjoy:** Transfer the cauliflower mash to a serving bowl. Serve hot, garnished with additional Parmesan cheese, chopped chives, or other desired toppings.

Cooking and Prep Time:

- Prep Time: 10 minutes
- Cook Time: 15-20 minutes

- Total Time: 25-30 minutes

Serving and Nutrition:

This recipe makes 4 servings of cauliflower mash.

Nutrition per serving (without Parmesan cheese):

- Calories: 100
- Total Fat: 6g
- Saturated Fat: 3g
- Cholesterol: 15mg
- Sodium: 150mg
- Total Carbohydrates: 9g
- Fiber: 3g
- Sugars: 4g
- Protein: 4g

5.3 Grilled Asparagus with Lemon

Ingredients:

- 1 lb asparagus, woody ends trimmed
- 2 tablespoons olive oil
- 1 tablespoon lemon juice
- 1 teaspoon lemon zest
- 1/4 teaspoon salt
- 1/4 teaspoon black pepper

Instructions:

1. **Prepare the Asparagus:** Trim the woody ends off the asparagus spears. You can do this by gently bending the asparagus near the bottom until it snaps naturally at the right spot.
2. **Make the Lemon Dressing:** In a small bowl, whisk together the olive oil, lemon juice, lemon zest, salt, and black pepper.
3. **Grill the Asparagus:** Preheat your grill or grill pan to medium-high heat. Place the asparagus spears on the grill in a single layer. Grill for 5-7 minutes, turning occasionally, until the asparagus is tender-crisp and has grill marks.
4. **Toss with Lemon Dressing:** Transfer the grilled asparagus to a serving dish. Drizzle the lemon dressing over the top and toss to coat the asparagus evenly.
5. **Serve:** Serve the grilled asparagus with lemon immediately, while still warm.

Cooking and Prep Time:

- Prep Time: 5 minutes
- Cook Time: 5-7 minutes
- Total Time: 10-12 minutes

Serving and Nutrition:

This recipe makes 4 servings.

Nutrition per serving:

- Calories: 80
- Total Fat: 6g
- Saturated Fat: 1g
- Cholesterol: 0mg
- Sodium: 150mg
- Total Carbohydrates: 6g
- Fiber: 3g
- Sugars: 2g
- Protein: 3g

5.4 Steamed Broccoli with Garlic

Ingredients:

- 1 lb broccoli florets
- 2 tablespoons olive oil
- 3 cloves garlic, minced
- 1/4 teaspoon salt
- 1/8 teaspoon black pepper

Instructions:

1. **Prepare the Broccoli:** Wash the broccoli florets and cut any large pieces into bite-sized florets.
2. **Steam the Broccoli:** Place the broccoli florets in a steamer basket set over a pot of simmering water. Cover and steam for 5-7 minutes, or until the broccoli is tender-crisp.
3. **Sauté the Garlic:** In a large skillet, heat the olive oil over medium heat. Add the minced garlic and sauté for 1-2 minutes, until fragrant.
4. **Toss with Broccoli:** Transfer the steamed broccoli to the skillet with the garlic. Toss to coat the broccoli evenly with the garlic and oil.
5. **Season and Serve:** Season the broccoli with salt and black pepper. Serve the steamed broccoli with garlic immediately, while hot.

Cooking and Prep Time:

- Prep Time: 5 minutes
- Cook Time: 7-9 minutes
- Total Time: 12-14 minutes

Serving and Nutrition:

This recipe makes 4 servings.

Nutrition per serving:

- Calories: 80
- Total Fat: 5g
- Saturated Fat: 1g
- Cholesterol: 0mg
- Sodium: 150mg
- Total Carbohydrates: 7g
- Fiber: 3g
- Sugars: 2g
- Protein: 3g

5.5 Roasted Sweet Potatoes

Ingredients:

- 2 lbs sweet potatoes, peeled and cut into 1-inch cubes
- 2 tablespoons olive oil
- 1 teaspoon ground cumin
- 1 teaspoon paprika
- 1/2 teaspoon garlic powder
- 1/2 teaspoon salt
- 1/4 teaspoon black pepper

Instructions:

1. Preheat your oven to 400°F (200°C).
2. In a large bowl, toss the cubed sweet potatoes with olive oil, cumin, paprika, garlic powder, salt, and black pepper until evenly coated.
3. Spread the seasoned sweet potato cubes in a single layer on a large baking sheet lined with parchment paper.
4. Roast for 25-30 minutes, flipping the potatoes halfway through, until they are tender and lightly browned on the edges.
5. Remove the roasted sweet potatoes from the oven and serve hot.

Cooking and Prep Time:

- Prep Time: 10 minutes
- Cook Time: 25-30 minutes
- Total Time: 35-40 minutes

Serving and Nutrition:

This recipe makes 4-6 servings.

Nutrition per serving (based on 6 servings):

- Calories: 150
- Total Fat: 5g
- Saturated Fat: 1g
- Cholesterol: 0mg
- Sodium: 260mg
- Total Carbohydrates: 25g
- Fiber: 4g
- Sugars: 7g
- Protein: 2g

5.6 Cucumber and Dill Salad

Ingredients:

- 2 large cucumbers, peeled and sliced into thin rounds
- 1/2 red onion, thinly sliced
- 1/4 cup fresh dill, chopped
- 1/4 cup white vinegar
- 2 tablespoons olive oil
- 1 tablespoon sugar
- 1 teaspoon salt
- 1/4 teaspoon black pepper

Instructions:

1. In a large bowl, combine the sliced cucumbers and red onion.
2. In a small bowl, whisk together the white vinegar, olive oil, sugar, salt, and black pepper until the sugar is dissolved.
3. Pour the dressing over the cucumbers and onions. Add the chopped fresh dill and toss gently to coat.
4. Cover and refrigerate for at least 30 minutes, or up to 2 hours, to allow the flavors to meld.
5. Serve chilled or at room temperature.

Cooking and Prep Time:

- Prep Time: 15 minutes
- Chilling Time: 30 minutes to 2 hours
- Total Time: 45 minutes to 2 hours 15 minutes

Serving and Nutrition:

This recipe makes 4-6 servings.

Nutrition per serving (based on 6 servings):

- Calories: 70
- Total Fat: 4g
- Saturated Fat: 0.5g
- Cholesterol: 0mg
- Sodium: 390mg
- Total Carbohydrates: 8g
- Fiber: 1g
- Sugars: 5g
- Protein: 1g

5.7 Balsamic Glazed Carrots

Ingredients:

- 1 lb carrots, peeled and cut into 1-inch pieces
- 2 tablespoons olive oil
- 2 tablespoons balsamic vinegar
- 1 tablespoon honey
- 1 clove garlic, minced
- 1/4 teaspoon salt
- 1/4 teaspoon black pepper

Instructions:

1. **Preheat the Oven:** Preheat your oven to 400°F (200°C).
2. **Prepare the Carrots:** Peel the carrots and cut them into 1-inch pieces.
3. **Make the Glaze:** In a small bowl, whisk together the olive oil, balsamic vinegar, honey, minced garlic, salt, and black pepper.
4. **Roast the Carrots:** Spread the carrot pieces in a single layer on a baking sheet. Drizzle the balsamic glaze over the carrots and toss to coat them evenly.
5. **Roast the Carrots:** Roast the carrots in the preheated oven for 20-25 minutes, stirring halfway, until they are tender and caramelized.
6. **Serve:** Transfer the balsamic glazed carrots to a serving dish and serve hot.

Cooking and Prep Time:

- Prep Time: 10 minutes
- Cook Time: 20-25 minutes
- Total Time: 30-35 minutes

Serving and Nutrition:

This recipe makes 4 servings.

Nutrition per serving:

- Calories: 120
- Total Fat: 5g
- Saturated Fat: 1g
- Cholesterol: 0mg
- Sodium: 230mg
- Total Carbohydrates: 18g
- Fiber: 3g
- Sugars: 11g
- Protein: 1g

5.8 Sautéed Spinach with Garlic

Ingredients:

- 1 lb fresh spinach, washed and stems removed
- 2 tablespoons olive oil
- 3 cloves garlic, minced
- 1/4 teaspoon salt
- 1/8 teaspoon black pepper

Instructions:

1. In a large skillet or wok, heat the olive oil over medium heat. Add the minced garlic and sauté for 1-2 minutes, until fragrant.
2. Add the fresh spinach to the skillet and toss to coat with the garlic oil. Season with salt and black pepper.
3. Cook the spinach, stirring frequently, for 2-3 minutes, until it is wilted and tender. Be careful not to overcook.
4. Remove the sautéed spinach from heat and serve immediately, while hot.

Cooking and Prep Time:

- Prep Time: 5 minutes
- Cook Time: 5 minutes
- Total Time: 10 minutes

Serving and Nutrition:

This recipe makes 4 servings.

Nutrition per serving:

- Calories: 70
- Total Fat: 5g
- Saturated Fat: 1g
- Cholesterol: 0mg

- Sodium: 260mg
- Total Carbohydrates: 5g
- Fiber: 3g
- Sugars: 0g
- Protein: 3g

5.9 Grilled Zucchini

Ingredients:

- 2 medium zucchinis, sliced lengthwise into 1/8-inch thick strips
- 2 tablespoons olive oil
- Salt and black pepper to taste
- Fresh herbs (optional, such as parsley or basil) for garnish

Instructions:

1. **Preheat the Grill:** Preheat your grill or grill pan to medium-high heat.
2. **Prepare the Zucchini:** Slice the zucchinis lengthwise into 1/8-inch thick strips.
3. **Brush with Oil:** Brush both sides of the zucchini slices with olive oil.
4. **Season:** Season the zucchini slices with salt and black pepper to taste.
5. **Grill:** Place the zucchini slices on the preheated grill. Grill for 2-3 minutes per side, or until they have grill marks and are tender.
6. **Serve:** Remove the grilled zucchini from the grill and serve hot, garnished with fresh herbs if desired.

Cooking and Prep Time:

- Prep Time: 5 minutes
- Cook Time: 4-6 minutes
- Total Time: 9-11 minutes

Serving and Nutrition:

This recipe makes 4 servings.

Nutrition per serving:

- Calories: 50
- Total Fat: 4g
- Saturated Fat: 1g
- Cholesterol: 0mg

- Sodium: 120mg
- Total Carbohydrates: 4g
- Fiber: 1g
- Sugars: 2g
- Protein: 1g

5.10 Tomato and Basil Salad

Ingredients:

- 3 cups cherry or grape tomatoes, halved
- 1 cup fresh basil leaves, chopped
- 2 tablespoons extra-virgin olive oil
- 1 tablespoon balsamic vinegar
- 1 teaspoon Dijon mustard
- 1/4 teaspoon salt
- 1/8 teaspoon black pepper

Instructions:

1. In a large bowl, combine the halved tomatoes and chopped basil leaves.
2. In a small bowl, whisk together the olive oil, balsamic vinegar, Dijon mustard, salt, and black pepper to make the dressing.
3. Pour the dressing over the tomatoes and basil, and gently toss to coat.
4. Let the salad sit for 5-10 minutes to allow the flavors to meld.
5. Serve the tomato and basil salad chilled or at room temperature.

Cooking and Prep Time:

- Prep Time: 10 minutes
- Total Time: 15-20 minutes

Serving and Nutrition:

This recipe makes 4 servings.

Nutrition per serving:

- Calories: 90
- Total Fat: 7g
- Saturated Fat: 1g
- Cholesterol: 0mg
- Sodium: 220mg

- Total Carbohydrates: 7g
- Fiber: 2g
- Sugars: 5g
- Protein: 2g

5.11 Quinoa Pilaf with Herbs

Ingredients:

- 1 cup quinoa, rinsed
- 2 cups vegetable broth
- 1 tablespoon olive oil
- 1 onion, diced
- 2 cloves garlic, minced
- 1 cup diced mushrooms
- 1/2 cup diced bell pepper
- 1/4 cup chopped fresh parsley
- 2 tablespoons chopped fresh basil
- 1 tablespoon chopped fresh thyme
- Salt and black pepper to taste

Instructions:

1. In a medium saucepan, combine the rinsed quinoa and vegetable broth. Bring to a boil over high heat.
2. Once boiling, reduce the heat to low, cover, and simmer for 15-20 minutes, or until the quinoa is tender and the liquid is absorbed.
3. Remove the quinoa from heat and fluff with a fork. Set aside.
4. In a large skillet, heat the olive oil over medium heat. Add the diced onion and sauté for 3-4 minutes, until translucent.
5. Add the minced garlic and continue cooking for 1 minute, until fragrant.
6. Stir in the diced mushrooms and bell pepper. Cook for 5-7 minutes, until the vegetables are tender.
7. Add the cooked quinoa to the skillet with the vegetables. Stir in the chopped parsley, basil, and thyme.
8. Season the quinoa pilaf with salt and black pepper to taste.

9. Serve the quinoa pilaf warm, as a side dish to your favorite protein or vegetarian main course.

Cooking and Prep Time:

- Prep Time: 10 minutes
- Cook Time: 20-25 minutes
- Total Time: 30-35 minutes

Serving and Nutrition:

This recipe makes 4 servings.

Nutrition per serving:

- Calories: 200
- Total Fat: 7g
- Saturated Fat: 1g
- Cholesterol: 0mg
- Sodium: 450mg
- Total Carbohydrates: 28g
- Fiber: 4g
- Sugars: 3g
- Protein: 7g

5.12 Spicy Roasted Cauliflower

Ingredients:

- 1 large head cauliflower, broken into evenly sized florets
- ¼ to ⅓ cup olive oil (or aquafaba for oil-free)
- 2 teaspoons smoked paprika (or chipotle powder)
- 3 tablespoons chili powder (American style)
- 2 teaspoons ground cumin
- 2 teaspoons garlic powder
- 2 teaspoons onion powder
- 1 teaspoon cayenne pepper
- ½ teaspoon black pepper
- 1 teaspoon salt

Instructions:

1. **Preheat the Oven:** Preheat your oven to 425°F (220°C).
2. **Prepare the Cauliflower:** Scatter the cauliflower florets onto a very large baking tray or use two medium-sized ones. Ensure there is enough room for the florets to be spread out in a single layer.
3. **Drizzle with Oil:** Drizzle the olive oil (or aquafaba) over the cauliflower florets. Using your hands, toss the florets to coat them evenly.
4. **Add Spices:** Sprinkle the smoked paprika, chili powder, cumin, garlic powder, onion powder, cayenne pepper, black pepper, and salt over the florets. Using your hands, toss and rub the spices into the florets until they are well coated.
5. **Roast the Cauliflower:** Bake the cauliflower in the top half of the oven for 25 minutes. Remove the tray from the oven and give the florets a good toss around, scraping up the oily spices from the bottom.
6. **Finish Cooking:** Return the tray to the oven and bake for an additional 20-30 minutes, until the cauliflower is sizzling, caramelized, and charred in places.
7. **Serve:** Remove the spicy roasted cauliflower from the oven and serve hot.

Cooking and Prep Time:

- Prep Time: 10 minutes
- Cook Time: 45-55 minutes
- Total Time: 55-65 minutes

Serving and Nutrition:

This recipe makes 4 servings.

Nutrition per serving:

- Calories: 164
- Total Fat: 14g
- Saturated Fat: 1g
- Cholesterol: 0mg
- Sodium: 629mg
- Total Carbohydrates: 8g
- Fiber: 3g
- Sugars: 2g
- Protein: 3g

5.13 Avocado and Lime Slaw

Ingredients:

- 1 medium head green cabbage, shredded (about 4 cups)
- 1 medium head red cabbage, shredded (about 4 cups)
- 1 large avocado, pitted and diced
- 1/4 cup freshly squeezed lime juice (about 2-3 limes)
- 2 tablespoons olive oil
- 1 teaspoon honey
- 1/2 teaspoon salt
- 1/4 teaspoon black pepper
- 2 tablespoons chopped fresh cilantro (optional)

Instructions:

1. In a large bowl, combine the shredded green and red cabbage.
2. In a small bowl, mash the diced avocado with a fork until it forms a creamy dressing-like consistency.
3. Whisk in the lime juice, olive oil, honey, salt, and black pepper until well combined.
4. Pour the avocado-lime dressing over the shredded cabbage and toss gently to coat.
5. Sprinkle the chopped fresh cilantro over the slaw, if using.
6. Cover and refrigerate the slaw for at least 30 minutes to allow the flavors to meld.
7. Serve the chilled avocado and lime slaw as a side dish.

Cooking and Prep Time:

- Prep Time: 15 minutes
- Chilling Time: 30 minutes
- Total Time: 45 minutes

Serving and Nutrition:

This recipe makes 6-8 servings.

Nutrition per serving (based on 6 servings):

- Calories: 160
- Total Fat: 11g
- Saturated Fat: 2g
- Cholesterol: 0mg
- Sodium: 260mg
- Total Carbohydrates: 16g
- Fiber: 6g
- Sugars: 6g
- Protein: 3g

5.14 Herb-Roasted Mushrooms

Ingredients:

- 1 lb mushrooms (such as cremini or button), cleaned and halved or quartered if large
- 2 tablespoons olive oil
- 2 cloves garlic, minced
- 1 tablespoon fresh thyme leaves
- 1 tablespoon fresh rosemary, chopped
- 1/2 teaspoon salt
- 1/4 teaspoon black pepper

Instructions:

1. Preheat your oven to 400°F (200°C).
2. In a large bowl, combine the halved or quartered mushrooms, olive oil, minced garlic, thyme leaves, chopped rosemary, salt, and black pepper. Toss until the mushrooms are evenly coated.
3. Spread the seasoned mushrooms in a single layer on a large baking sheet lined with parchment paper.
4. Roast the mushrooms for 15-20 minutes, stirring halfway, until they are tender and lightly browned.
5. Remove the herb-roasted mushrooms from the oven and serve hot, garnished with additional fresh thyme or rosemary if desired.

Cooking and Prep Time:

- Prep Time: 10 minutes
- Cook Time: 15-20 minutes
- Total Time: 25-30 minutes

Serving and Nutrition:

This recipe makes 4 servings.

Nutrition per serving:

- Calories: 100
- Total Fat: 7g
- Saturated Fat: 1g
- Cholesterol: 0mg
- Sodium: 300mg
- Total Carbohydrates: 7g
- Fiber: 2g
- Sugars: 2g
- Protein: 3g

5.15 Fresh Green Bean Salad

Ingredients:

- 1 lb fresh green beans, trimmed and cut into 1-inch pieces
- 1 red bell pepper, diced
- 1 cup cherry tomatoes, halved
- 1/2 red onion, thinly sliced
- 1/4 cup chopped fresh parsley
- 2 tablespoons chopped fresh basil
- 2 tablespoons olive oil
- 2 tablespoons red wine vinegar
- 1 tablespoon Dijon mustard
- 1 garlic clove, minced
- 1/2 teaspoon salt
- 1/4 teaspoon black pepper

Instructions:

1. **Blanch the Green Beans:** Bring a large pot of salted water to a boil. Add the trimmed and cut green beans and cook for 2-3 minutes, until crisp-tender. Drain the beans and immediately transfer them to an ice bath to stop the cooking process. Drain the beans again and pat them dry.
2. **Make the Dressing:** In a small bowl, whisk together the olive oil, red wine vinegar, Dijon mustard, minced garlic, salt, and black pepper.
3. **Assemble the Salad:** In a large bowl, combine the blanched green beans, diced red bell pepper, halved cherry tomatoes, sliced red onion, chopped parsley, and chopped basil.
4. **Toss with Dressing:** Pour the dressing over the salad and toss gently to coat the vegetables evenly.
5. **Chill and Serve:** Cover the salad and refrigerate for at least 30 minutes to allow the flavors to meld. Serve chilled or at room temperature.

Cooking and Prep Time:

- Prep Time: 15 minutes
- Cook Time: 3 minutes
- Chilling Time: 30 minutes
- Total Time: 48 minutes

Serving and Nutrition:

This recipe makes 6 servings.

Nutrition per serving:

- Calories: 110
- Total Fat: 6g
- Saturated Fat: 1g
- Cholesterol: 0mg
- Sodium: 260mg
- Total Carbohydrates: 12g
- Fiber: 4g
- Sugars: 5g
- Protein: 3g

Chapter:6 Dessert Recipes

6.1 Mixed Berry Sorbet

Ingredients:

- 2 cups mixed berries (such as raspberries, blackberries, and blueberries)
- 1/2 cup granulated sugar
- 2 tablespoons lemon juice
- 1 tablespoon water

Instructions:

1. **Prepare the Berry Purée:** In a medium saucepan, combine the mixed berries, sugar, lemon juice, and water. Bring the mixture to a simmer over medium heat, stirring occasionally, until the sugar has dissolved and the berries have softened, about 5-7 minutes.
2. **Blend the Mixture:** Transfer the berry mixture to a blender and blend until smooth. Strain the purée through a fine-mesh sieve to remove any seeds or pulp, if desired.
3. **Chill the Mixture:** Pour the strained berry purée into a shallow baking dish or metal pan. Cover and refrigerate for at least 2 hours, or until completely chilled.
4. **Freeze the Sorbet:** Once the berry mixture is thoroughly chilled, transfer it to an ice cream maker and churn according to the manufacturer's instructions, usually 20-30 minutes.
5. **Serve:** Scoop the mixed berry sorbet into serving dishes and enjoy immediately. If the sorbet has become too firm, let it sit at room temperature for 5-10 minutes before scooping.

Cooking and Prep Time:

- Prep Time: 15 minutes
- Chilling Time: 2 hours

- Churning Time: 20-30 minutes
- Total Time: 2 hours 35 minutes - 2 hours 45 minutes

Serving and Nutrition:

This recipe makes approximately 4 servings.

Nutrition per serving:

- Calories: 130
- Total Fat: 0g
- Saturated Fat: 0g
- Cholesterol: 0mg
- Sodium: 5mg
- Total Carbohydrates: 33g
- Fiber: 4g
- Sugars: 29g
- Protein: 1g

6.2 Baked Apples with Cinnamon

Ingredients:

- 4-6 medium apples (such as Honeycrisp, Gala, or Fuji), peeled, cored, and sliced into 1/2-inch thick wedges
- 1/4 cup packed brown sugar
- 1 tablespoon ground cinnamon
- 1 tablespoon unsalted butter, cut into small pieces
- 1 tablespoon lemon juice
- 1/4 cup chopped walnuts or pecans (optional)

Instructions:

1. **Preheat the Oven:** Preheat your oven to 375°F (190°C).
2. **Prepare the Apples:** Peel, core, and slice the apples into 1/2-inch thick wedges. Place the apple slices in a large bowl.
3. **Make the Cinnamon-Sugar Mixture:** In a small bowl, mix together the brown sugar and ground cinnamon until well combined.
4. **Toss the Apples:** Add the cinnamon-sugar mixture to the bowl with the apple slices. Toss gently to coat the apples evenly.
5. **Assemble the Dish:** Transfer the cinnamon-sugar coated apple slices to a 9x13-inch baking dish. Dot the top of the apples with the pieces of unsalted butter.
6. **Bake the Apples:** Cover the baking dish with aluminum foil and bake for 30 minutes. Remove the foil and continue baking for an additional 15-20 minutes, or until the apples are tender and the juices are bubbling.
7. **Finish and Serve:** Remove the baked apples from the oven and drizzle the lemon juice over the top. Sprinkle the chopped walnuts or pecans over the apples, if using.
8. **Serve Warm:** Serve the baked apples warm, either on their own or with a scoop of vanilla ice cream.

Cooking and Prep Time:

- Prep Time: 15 minutes
- Cook Time: 45-50 minutes
- Total Time: 1 hour

Serving and Nutrition:

This recipe makes 4-6 servings.

Nutrition per serving (based on 6 servings):

- Calories: 180
- Total Fat: 6g
- Saturated Fat: 2g
- Cholesterol: 5mg
- Sodium: 0mg
- Total Carbohydrates: 34g
- Fiber: 4g
- Sugars: 26g
- Protein: 1g

6.3 Chia Seed Pudding

Ingredients:

- 1/4 cup chia seeds
- 1 cup milk (dairy, almond, coconut, etc.)
- 2-3 tablespoons maple syrup, honey, or other sweetener (adjust to taste)
- 1/2 teaspoon vanilla extract (optional)
- Toppings (such as fresh fruit, nuts, coconut, cinnamon)

Instructions:

1. **Combine the Ingredients:** In a medium bowl or mason jar, whisk together the chia seeds, milk, sweetener, and vanilla (if using) until well combined.
2. **Chill and Let Set:** Cover the bowl or seal the jar and refrigerate for at least 2 hours, or up to 5 days. The chia seeds will absorb the liquid and thicken the pudding as it chills.
3. **Add Toppings:** When ready to serve, give the chia pudding a stir and top with your desired toppings, such as fresh fruit, nuts, coconut, or a sprinkle of cinnamon.

Cooking and Prep Time:

- Prep Time: 5 minutes
- Chilling Time: 2 hours (minimum)
- Total Time: 2 hours 5 minutes

Serving and Nutrition:

This recipe makes 2 servings.

Nutrition per serving (using 1 cup of unsweetened almond milk and 2 tablespoons of maple syrup):

- Calories: 200
- Total Fat: 9g

- Saturated Fat: 1g
- Cholesterol: 0mg
- Sodium: 75mg
- Total Carbohydrates: 25g
- Fiber: 9g
- Sugars: 14g
- Protein: 6g

6.4 Fresh Fruit Kabobs

Ingredients:

- 3 bananas, cut into 1-inch chunks
- 2 cups pineapple chunks (30-40 pieces)
- 30-40 strawberries
- 30-40 seedless grapes
- 1/2 cup orange juice
- 10 wooden skewers
- Apple jelly (optional)

Instructions:

1. **Prepare the Fruit:** Cut the bananas into 1-inch chunks. Combine the orange juice with the banana chunks and gently toss to coat the bananas.
2. **Thread the Fruit:** Take a wooden skewer and thread the cut-up bananas, pineapple chunks, strawberries, and seedless grapes onto the skewer.
3. **Enhance the Sweetness:** If using, slice the strawberries in half and place them in a medium bowl. Add a bit of sugar and toss to coat the strawberries. This method enhances the sweetness of the strawberries.
4. **Add Apple Jelly (Optional):** If using apple jelly, add about 5 large tablespoons to a small saucepan. Stir over medium heat until the jelly becomes less lumpy. Let it cool.
5. **Coat the Fruit:** Slice the bananas and coat them with apple jelly. Slice the strawberries and cut them in half. Coat the sliced strawberries with either sugar or apple jelly.
6. **Assemble the Kabobs:** Stick the fruit on the skewers.
7. **Serve:** Enjoy the fresh fruit kabobs immediately.

Cooking and Prep Time:

- Prep Time: 15 minutes
- Total Time: 15 minutes

Serving and Nutrition:

This recipe makes 10 servings.

Nutrition per serving (based on 10 servings):

- Calories: 180
- Total Fat: 0g
- Saturated Fat: 0g
- Cholesterol: 0mg
- Sodium: 0mg
- Total Carbohydrates: 45g
- Fiber: 4g
- Sugars: 34g
- Protein: 2g

6.5 Banana Nice Cream

Ingredients:

- 3-4 ripe bananas, peeled and frozen
- 1/4 cup milk (dairy, almond, or coconut)
- 1 tablespoon peanut butter or other nut butter (optional)
- 1 teaspoon vanilla extract (optional)
- Toppings (such as fresh fruit, nuts, chocolate chips, or shredded coconut)

Instructions:

1. **Freeze the Bananas:** Peel the ripe bananas and place them in a single layer on a baking sheet lined with parchment paper. Freeze for at least 2 hours, or until completely frozen.
2. **Blend the Ingredients:** In a high-powered blender or food processor, combine the frozen bananas, milk, peanut butter (if using), and vanilla extract (if using). Blend until smooth and creamy, scraping down the sides as needed.
3. **Serve:** Scoop the banana nice cream into bowls or cups. Top with your desired toppings, such as fresh fruit, nuts, chocolate chips, or shredded coconut.
4. **Freeze:** If the nice cream becomes too soft, place it back in the freezer for 10-15 minutes before serving.

Cooking and Prep Time:

- Prep Time: 10 minutes
- Freezing Time: 2 hours
- Total Time: 2 hours 10 minutes

Serving and Nutrition:

This recipe makes approximately 4 servings.

Nutrition per serving (without toppings):

- Calories: 100

- Total Fat: 1g
- Saturated Fat: 0g
- Cholesterol: 0mg
- Sodium: 0mg
- Total Carbohydrates: 23g
- Fiber: 3g
- Sugars: 12g
- Protein: 1g

6.6 Watermelon Granita

Ingredients:

- 4 cups cubed seedless watermelon (about 1 medium watermelon)
- 1/4 cup granulated sugar
- 2 tablespoons fresh lime juice

Instructions:

1. **Freeze the Watermelon:** Cut the watermelon into 1-inch cubes and place them in a single layer on a baking sheet. Freeze for at least 2 hours, or until completely frozen.
2. **Make the Granita Mixture:** In a blender or food processor, combine the frozen watermelon cubes, sugar, and lime juice. Blend until smooth and the sugar has dissolved.
3. **Freeze and Scrape:** Pour the watermelon mixture into a shallow baking dish or metal pan. Place in the freezer and let it freeze for 1 hour.
4. **Scrape the Granita:** Using a fork, scrape the partially frozen mixture to create icy flakes. Return the pan to the freezer and repeat the scraping process every 30 minutes until the granita is fully frozen and has a crunchy, icy texture, about 2-3 hours total.
5. **Serve:** Scoop the watermelon granita into glasses or bowls and serve immediately. Garnish with fresh mint leaves, if desired.

Cooking and Prep Time:

- Prep Time: 10 minutes
- Freezing Time: 2-3 hours
- Total Time: 2 hours 10 minutes - 3 hours 10 minutes

Serving and Nutrition:

This recipe makes approximately 4 servings.

Nutrition per serving:

- Calories: 100
- Total Fat: 0g
- Saturated Fat: 0g
- Cholesterol: 0mg
- Sodium: 0mg
- Total Carbohydrates: 26g
- Fiber: 1g
- Sugars: 24g
- Protein: 1g

6.7 Mango Coconut Smoothie

Ingredients:

- 2 cups frozen mango chunks
- 1 cup unsweetened coconut milk (from a can or carton)
- 1/4 cup plain Greek yogurt (or coconut yogurt)
- 2 tablespoons honey (or maple syrup)
- 1/2 teaspoon vanilla extract
- Pinch of salt

Instructions:

1. **Blend the Ingredients:** In a high-powered blender, combine the frozen mango chunks, coconut milk, Greek yogurt, honey, vanilla extract, and a pinch of salt. Blend on high speed until the mixture is smooth and creamy.
2. **Adjust Sweetness:** Taste the smoothie and adjust the sweetness by adding more honey or maple syrup if desired.
3. **Serve:** Pour the mango coconut smoothie into glasses and serve immediately. Garnish with a slice of fresh mango or a sprinkle of toasted coconut, if desired.

Cooking and Prep Time:

- Prep Time: 5 minutes
- Blending Time: 2-3 minutes
- Total Time: 7-8 minutes

Serving and Nutrition:

This recipe makes 2 servings.

Nutrition per serving:

- Calories: 270
- Total Fat: 13g
- Saturated Fat: 11g

- Cholesterol: 5mg
- Sodium: 45mg
- Total Carbohydrates: 35g
- Fiber: 3g
- Sugars: 29g
- Protein: 5g

6.8 Poached Pears with Vanilla

Ingredients:

- 4 ripe pears, peeled and halved
- 1 cup water
- 1/2 cup granulated sugar
- 1/2 vanilla bean, split lengthwise
- 1/4 cup fresh lemon juice
- 1/4 cup fresh orange juice
- 1/4 cup fresh thyme leaves (optional)

Instructions:

1. **Prepare the Syrup:** In a large saucepan, combine the water, granulated sugar, and the split vanilla bean. Bring the mixture to a boil over medium-high heat, stirring occasionally to dissolve the sugar.
2. **Add the Pears:** Add the peeled and halved pears to the boiling syrup. Reduce the heat to medium-low and simmer the pears for 20-25 minutes, or until they are tender and easily pierced with a fork.
3. **Add Lemon and Orange Juice:** Remove the pears from the heat and add the lemon juice and orange juice. Stir to combine.
4. **Cool and Serve:** Let the pears cool in the syrup for at least 30 minutes. Serve the pears warm or chilled, garnished with fresh thyme leaves if desired.

Cooking and Prep Time:

- Prep Time: 10 minutes
- Cooking Time: 20-25 minutes
- Total Time: 35-40 minutes

Serving and Nutrition:

This recipe makes 4 servings.

Nutrition per serving:

- Calories: 150
- Total Fat: 0g
- Saturated Fat: 0g
- Cholesterol: 0mg
- Sodium: 10mg
- Total Carbohydrates: 35g
- Fiber: 4g
- Sugars: 28g

6.9 Strawberry Banana Sorbet

Ingredients:

- 2 cups fresh strawberries, hulled and sliced
- 2 ripe bananas, peeled and sliced
- 2 tablespoons honey (or maple syrup)
- 1 tablespoon fresh lemon juice

Instructions:

1. **Freeze the Fruit:** Arrange the sliced strawberries and banana pieces in a single layer on a baking sheet. Freeze for at least 2 hours, or until completely frozen.
2. **Make the Sorbet:** In a food processor or high-powered blender, combine the frozen strawberries, frozen banana slices, honey, and lemon juice. Blend until smooth and creamy, scraping down the sides as needed.
3. **Freeze and Serve:** Transfer the strawberry banana sorbet mixture to a freezer-safe container. Cover and freeze for 2-3 hours, stirring every 30 minutes, until the sorbet reaches your desired consistency.
4. **Serve:** Scoop the strawberry banana sorbet into bowls or cups and serve immediately. Garnish with fresh strawberry slices, if desired.

Cooking and Prep Time:

- Prep Time: 15 minutes
- Freezing Time: 4-5 hours
- Total Time: 4 hours 15 minutes

Serving and Nutrition:

This recipe makes approximately 4 servings.
Nutrition per serving:

- Calories: 120
- Total Fat: 0g

- Saturated Fat: 0g
- Cholesterol: 0mg
- Sodium: 0mg
- Total Carbohydrates: 30g
- Fiber: 3g
- Sugars: 20g
- Protein: 1g

6.10 Pineapple Coconut Whip

Ingredients:

- 1 can (20 oz) crushed pineapple, drained
- 1 can (14 oz) coconut cream
- 1/2 cup powdered sugar
- 1/4 teaspoon salt
- 1/4 teaspoon vanilla extract
- 1/4 cup shredded coconut (optional)

Instructions:

1. **Drain the Pineapple:** Drain the crushed pineapple in a fine-mesh sieve to remove excess liquid.
2. **Whip the Coconut Cream:** In a large bowl, whip the coconut cream until it forms stiff peaks.
3. **Add the Pineapple:** Gently fold the drained pineapple into the whipped coconut cream.
4. **Add the Sugar and Salt:** Add the powdered sugar and salt to the pineapple-coconut mixture and fold until well combined.
5. **Add Vanilla and Shredded Coconut (Optional):** Add the vanilla extract and shredded coconut (if using) and fold until well combined.
6. **Serve:** Spoon the pineapple coconut whip into serving bowls or cups and serve immediately.

Cooking and Prep Time:

- Prep Time: 10 minutes
- Total Time: 10 minutes

Serving and Nutrition:

This recipe makes approximately 4 servings.

Nutrition per serving:

- Calories: 150
- Total Fat: 12g
- Saturated Fat: 10g
- Cholesterol: 0mg
- Sodium: 45mg
- Total Carbohydrates: 15g
- Fiber: 1g
- Sugars: 12g
- Protein: 1g

6.11 Raspberry Lemonade Popsicles

Ingredients:

- 1 1/2 cups lemonade (homemade or store-bought)
- 1/2 cup fresh raspberries
- Popsicle mold and sticks

Instructions:

1. Place a few raspberries in the bottom of each popsicle mold cavity. Gently push them down with a spoon or popsicle stick to keep them in place once the lemonade is added.
2. Slowly fill the mold cavities about 3/4 full with lemonade. Push any floating raspberries back into place. Add a few more raspberries to each cavity.
3. Place the filled mold in the freezer for 1-1.5 hours. Once the tops are icy, insert the popsicle sticks and freeze for an additional 4-6 hours, until completely set.
4. To remove the popsicles, run the mold under warm water for a few seconds. Gently pull on the sticks to release the popsicles from the mold.

Cooking and Prep Time:

- Prep Time: 10 minutes
- Freezing Time: 5-7.5 hours
- Total Time: 5 hours 10 minutes

Serving and Nutrition:

This recipe makes approximately 6 popsicles.

Nutrition per serving (1 popsicle):

- Calories: 30
- Total Fat: 0g
- Saturated Fat: 0g
- Cholesterol: 0mg

- Sodium: 0mg
- Total Carbohydrates: 7g
- Fiber: 1g
- Sugars: 6g
- Protein: 0g

6.12 Grilled Peaches with Honey

Ingredients:

- 4 ripe but firm peaches, halved and pitted
- 2 tablespoons olive oil or melted butter
- 1/4 cup honey
- 1 tablespoon fresh lemon juice
- 1/2 teaspoon ground cinnamon (optional)
- Vanilla ice cream or whipped cream (optional, for serving)

Instructions:

1. **Preheat the Grill:** Preheat your grill or grill pan to medium-high heat.
2. **Prepare the Peaches:** Halve the peaches and remove the pits. Brush the cut sides of the peach halves with the olive oil or melted butter.
3. **Grill the Peaches:** Place the peach halves, cut-side down, on the preheated grill. Grill for 4-6 minutes, or until the peaches are softened and have grill marks on the cut side.
4. **Flip and Finish Grilling:** Carefully flip the peach halves and grill for an additional 2-3 minutes, or until the peaches are tender and slightly charred.
5. **Make the Honey Drizzle:** In a small bowl, whisk together the honey and lemon juice.
6. **Serve:** Transfer the grilled peach halves to a serving plate. Drizzle the honey mixture over the top and sprinkle with ground cinnamon, if desired. Serve the grilled peaches warm, with a scoop of vanilla ice cream or a dollop of whipped cream, if desired.

Cooking and Prep Time:

- Prep Time: 10 minutes
- Grilling Time: 6-9 minutes
- Total Time: 16-19 minutes

Serving and Nutrition:

This recipe makes 4 servings (2 peach halves per serving).

Nutrition per serving (without ice cream or whipped cream):

- Calories: 150
- Total Fat: 5g
- Saturated Fat: 1g
- Cholesterol: 0mg
- Sodium: 0mg
- Total Carbohydrates: 28g
- Fiber: 2g
- Sugars: 24g
- Protein: 1g

6.13 Kiwi and Lime Sorbet

Ingredients:

- 4 ripe kiwi fruits, peeled and chopped
- 1/2 cup freshly squeezed lime juice (about 4-5 limes)
- 1/2 cup granulated sugar
- 1/4 cup water

Instructions:

1. **Prepare the Kiwi Purée:** In a blender or food processor, blend the chopped kiwi fruit until smooth. Strain the purée through a fine-mesh sieve to remove any seeds or pulp.
2. **Make the Sorbet Base:** In a small saucepan, combine the granulated sugar and water. Bring the mixture to a boil, stirring occasionally, until the sugar has fully dissolved. Remove from heat and let cool completely.
3. **Combine the Ingredients:** In a medium bowl, whisk together the kiwi purée, lime juice, and the cooled sugar syrup until well combined.
4. **Freeze the Sorbet:** Pour the kiwi-lime mixture into a shallow baking dish or metal pan. Place in the freezer and stir the mixture with a fork every 30 minutes for the first 2 hours, until it starts to freeze around the edges.
5. **Finish Freezing:** Continue freezing the sorbet, stirring every 30-60 minutes, until it reaches your desired consistency, about 3-4 hours total.
6. **Serve:** Scoop the kiwi and lime sorbet into bowls or glasses and serve immediately. Garnish with a slice of kiwi or a lime wedge, if desired.

Cooking and Prep Time:

- Prep Time: 15 minutes
- Freezing Time: 3-4 hours
- Total Time: 3 hours 15 minutes - 4 hours 15 minutes

Serving and Nutrition:

This recipe makes approximately 4 servings.

Nutrition per serving:

- Calories: 130
- Total Fat: 0g
- Saturated Fat: 0g
- Cholesterol: 0mg
- Sodium: 0mg
- Total Carbohydrates: 33g
- Fiber: 2g
- Sugars: 30g
- Protein: 1g

6.14 Apple Cranberry Compote

Ingredients:

- 2 cups peeled, cored, and diced apples (about 2 medium apples)
- 1 cup fresh or frozen cranberries
- 1/4 cup granulated sugar
- 1/4 cup water
- 1 teaspoon ground cinnamon
- 1/4 teaspoon ground nutmeg
- 1/4 teaspoon salt

Instructions:

1. In a medium saucepan, combine the diced apples, cranberries, sugar, water, cinnamon, nutmeg, and salt.
2. Bring the mixture to a boil over medium heat, stirring occasionally.
3. Once boiling, reduce the heat to low and let the compote simmer for 15-20 minutes, stirring occasionally, until the apples are tender and the cranberries have burst.
4. Remove the compote from heat and let it cool slightly before serving.

Cooking and Prep Time:

- Prep Time: 10 minutes
- Cook Time: 15-20 minutes
- Total Time: 25-30 minutes

Serving and Nutrition:

This recipe makes approximately 4 servings.

Nutrition per serving (1/4 of the recipe):

- Calories: 120
- Total Fat: 0g
- Saturated Fat: 0g

- Cholesterol: 0mg
- Sodium: 120mg
- Total Carbohydrates: 31g
- Fiber: 4g
- Sugars: 25g
- Protein: 0g

6.15 Blueberry Lemon Parfait

Ingredients:

- 2 cups fresh blueberries
- 1/2 cup lemon curd
- 2 cups plain Greek yogurt
- 2 tablespoons honey (optional)
- Lemon zest for garnish (optional)

Instructions:

1. **Prepare the Lemon Curd:** If you don't have pre-made lemon curd, you can make your own by following a simple recipe. Alternatively, you can use store-bought lemon curd.
2. **Assemble the Parfait:** In a clear glass or parfait dish, layer the ingredients in the following order:1/4 cup blueberries
- ❖ 2 tablespoons lemon curd
- ❖ 1/2 cup Greek yogurt
- ❖ Repeat the layers until you reach the top of the glass, ending with a layer of yogurt
3. **Chill and Serve:** Refrigerate the parfaits for at least 30 minutes to allow the flavors to meld.
4. **Garnish and Serve:** Just before serving, drizzle a bit of honey over the top of the parfait (if desired) and sprinkle with lemon zest.

Cooking and Prep Time:

- Prep Time: 10 minutes
- Chilling Time: 30 minutes
- Total Time: 40 minutes

Serving and Nutrition:

This recipe makes 4 servings.

Nutrition per serving:

- Calories: 180
- Total Fat: 3g
- Saturated Fat: 1g
- Cholesterol: 15mg
- Sodium: 55mg
- Total Carbohydrates: 31g
- Fiber: 3g
- Sugars: 24g
- Protein: 10g

www.ingramcontent.com/pod-product-compliance
Lightning Source LLC
Chambersburg PA
CBHW081434250726
48662CB00009B/2782